Phyllis Speight studied the philosophy and materia medica of Homoeopathy for four years before going into partnership with Noel Puddephatt. They practised first in Brighton and then in London. When Mr Puddephatt went abroad, Phyllis Speight continued to work in London, and expanded her practice to include first Hampshire and then Sussex.

In December 1974 she and her husband moved to Devonshire to retire, but at her patients' request she started working again. Apart from contributing articles to magazines and journals, she is also the author of several other authoritative works on Homoeopathy.

Phyllis Speight

Homoeopathy

A Practical Guide to Natural Medicine

A MAYFLOWER BOOK

GRANADA

London Toronto Sydney New York

Published by Granada Publishing Limited in 1979
Reprinted in 1982

ISBN 0 583 12907 2

A Mayflower UK original

Granada Publishing Limited
Frogmore, St Albans, Herts AL2 2NF
and
36 Golden Square, London W1R 4AH
866 United Nations Plaza, New York, NY 10017, USA
117 York Street, Sydney, NSW 2000, Australia
100 Skyway Avenue, Rexdale, Ontario, M9W 3A6, Canada
61 Beach Road, Auckland, New Zealand

Set, printed and bound in Great Britain by
Cox & Wyman Ltd, Reading
Set in Intertype Times

Contents

Foreword

'Homoeopathy – the most complete and scientific system of healing the world has ever seen'

John H. Clarke, MD

The wind of change is blowing through the world of healing with considerable force. The man in the street is becoming more and more discontented with drug therapy and conscious that it leaves much to be desired. Public awareness of the value of 'fringe' medicine is increasing through television, articles in the press and many books published each year.

The basis of homoeopathy is rational in that it treats the whole man rather than his parts and there are no side effects from homoeopathic remedies.

I sincerely hope that this book will bring the benefits of homoeopathy to the notice of a much wider public.

Phyllis Speight
Devon 1977

Introduction

The general public have, as a rule, but one criterion for judging worth, and this is well expressed in the proverb 'The proof of the pudding is in the eating' – that is to say, once satisfied with results they ask no questions as to why and wherefore; and even among earnest, thoughtful people, the full occupation of their energy in the battle of life precludes very much thinking beyond certain established lines.

Have *you* ever pondered the subject of medicine today? Many people grumble about the side effects of drugs and often I hear 'My doctors says I have to live with it', but what are the deeper implications of this?

No botanist has discovered the power inherent in seed or bulb which determines the colour of the flower, either by microscope or spectrum tests. Yet no one can deny that 'something' must be inherent in the cells of the seed or bulb which determines and fixes the colour.

A daughter gets a wart just above her eyebrow in her 13th year. The father had just such a wart in exactly the same place over the left eyebrow, which in his case appeared in his 14th year. The dermatologist might say that warts are merely a local condition of the skin. Would anyone accept as a reasonable explanation that this wart snowed down from the sky at this opportune time?

A person receives a blow upon the leg. At once nature begins the work of repair, removes injured tissue and puts in new, and the wound is healed. Another person receives the same sort or even a lesser injury. It does not heal but grows worse, and an ulcer forms to remain for months or years. Why? The difference cannot be explained mechanically but rather by what we shall call *vital force*. And so the difference between a person who withstands all kinds of exposure, climate and infections, and a person who catches everything he meets.

You can trace (by a process of careful reasoning and explanation) a trouble back to the liver as being the organ primarily at fault. But why does the liver not function properly? What makes it act harmoniously in health? *The vital stimulus within.* The primary fault is not the lesion in any organ, for a faultless vital force would prevent or quickly repair it; and even infectious germs cannot gain a hold where its action is perfect. If rheumatism sets in due to uric acid, one must introduce something to dissolve and eliminate this acid. But what is the cause of the uric acid? What eliminates it in health? Even if you trace it back to a certain organ or to a germ, the vital force is still basically responsible for that condition.

Yet there is nothing in orthodox medicine which comprehends this vital element in disease. Orthodox medicine considers only the organs, sees only the mechanical and pathological condition, and seeks to change that by direct action from without. If an organ is lax in its action, its activity is forced with a drug known to possess the capacity to do so, although it is evident that this will be followed by a reaction tending towards even greater sluggishness.

Now when we have removed any mechanical or other exciting, maintaining causes, corrected bad habits or abuse, and still a trouble remains, since that vital force controls absolutely vital action and repair, is it not clear that it is the vital force which is disturbed, overpowered, sick?

Orthodox medicine tries to force the organs to cure the man. But the man is not sick because his organs fail to act. They fail to act because *he is sick.* Then why not treat the man instead of his organs? – the whole man, the real man, the man behind the organs – and thus restore the natural action of organs and so secure the removal of disease matter and all those pathological states which are results and not causes?

Some physicians attempt to control *dynamic* derangements by mechanical or material means. But the dynamic element in disease can only be met by the dynamic element in the remedy.

The homoeopath does not prescribe only for the disease but for the sick individual as a whole. The prescription is not based upon a hypothetical diagnosis but upon the totality of the symptoms of the particular case, with due regard to its pathological classification. Of twenty cases of acute articular rheumatism, all may be cured and yet no two receive the same remedy, simply because under our method of examination it is found that no two cases present exactly the same aches and pains, or the same grouping of symptoms. It is true that all the cases may present the symptoms common to most cases of rheumatism – that is to say all may have pain, fever and swollen joints – but when these symptoms common to the diagnosis are set aside and we proceed to the further examination of the patient, we find that his remaining symptoms group themselves in an entirely personal manner. His case presents features quite as peculiar to him as are the markings on the ball of the thumb, which latter fact the Chinese discovered to be an absolutely identifying feature some thousands of years ago.

Manifestly, therefore, a truly effective method of healing the sick must be one which will enable the homoeopath to select a remedy required for the peculiar symptoms of the sick individual. The principles of classical homoeopathy call for the most painstaking examination and identification of case and remedy, and to this end individualization is absolutely necessary.

I have discussed these and other points in the following chapters. In Part Two I have given case histories illustrating the use of homoeopathy in a wide variety of cases.

PART ONE

Homoeopathy in Practice

CHAPTER 1

Christian Samuel Hahnemann

Samuel Hahnemann (as he is known) was born in Meissen in 1755 to educated parents who lived in poor circumstances. Botany, mathematics and geometry were the subjects the boy was most interested in, and it is on record that he made a herbarium when he was quite a small child. In addition to his studies at school, his father was wont to leave Samuel in a room on his own with a problem to work out in a given time. Thus the boy's mind and powers of concentration developed far more quickly than those of most other boys of his age.

His father was a painter of Dresden china for the Meissen pottery, but on the orders of Frederick II of Prussia the porcelain factory was raided and subsequently closed down. This meant that Samuel had to leave school and become an apprentice to a grocery store in Leipsic. It was fortunate that the rector of the school realized the potential of the young Hahnemann and persuaded his father to allow him to return without having to pay any fees. The rector took Samuel under his wing and the boy soon caught up and was able to assist younger scholars with their lessons in Greek. When he left school at the age of 20 he delivered a Latin Oration entitled 'The Wonderful Construction of the Human Hand'.

Hahnemann then went back to Leipsic to study medicine. He was still very poor, and to supplement the small allowance from his parents he taught French and German, as he was a brilliant linguist, and every third night he spent on translations. He left Leipsic for the most advanced medical school in Europe – Vienna. Before he qualified Hahnemann became family physician and librarian to the Governor of

Transylvania. Here he came into contact with ague, which was rife in the district, and by the time he left he had a thorough knowledge of the disease and the treatment for it. A medical degree was conferred on him in 1779.

In 1782 this young doctor, who was now working closely with an apothecary, married the latter's step-daughter, and soon afterwards was appointed Medical Officer of Health in Dessau. Hahnemann was by this time becoming more and more disillusioned with the medicine of his day, and by 1790 he was in despair. By then he had five children which meant he had a family of seven to support; so he gave up practising medicine and turned all his attentions to translating in order to bring in money.

And then Cullen's *Materia Medica* came into his hands to be translated. Despite the fact that Professor Cullen was an eminent Scottish physician, Hahnemann found that he could not agree with the explanation that Cullen gave about the action of quinine in the treatment of malaria (ague). He then decided to test the drug on himself, an experience which he described as follows:

> For the sake of experiment I took for several days four queurschen (drachms) of good cinchona twice a day. My feet, the tips of my fingers, etc., first became cold, and I felt tired and sleepy; then my heart began to beat, my pulse became hard and quick, got an insufferable feeling of uneasiness, a trembling (but without rigor), a weariness in all my limbs, then a beating in my head, redness of the cheeks, thirst; in short, all the old symptoms with which I was familiar in Ague appeared one after the other. Also, those particularly characteristic symptoms which I was wont to observe in Agues – obtuseness of the senses, a kind of stiffness in all the limbs, but especially that dull disagreeable feeling which seems to have its seat in the periosteum of all the bones in the body – these all put in an appearance. This paroxysm lasted each time for two or three hours, and came again afresh whenever I repeated the dose, not otherwise. I left off and I became well.

This simple experiment altered the whole of Hahnemann's medical thinking and consequently his future. It occurred to him that if this drug could produce similar symptoms to those of malaria it would also *cure* malaria. He had, in fact, stumbled on the Law of Similars, like will be cured by like – *Similia Similibus Curentur*, the foundation stone on which homoeopathy rests. The next six years Hahnemann spent patiently experimenting and observing. At last he was convinced that treatment should be by substances which, when taken in material doses, could produce in healthy people symptoms similar to those characteristic of the disease to be treated. He now felt that he could practise this new form of medicine and he returned to Leipsic. But he continued to investigate more and more drugs by testing them on his family and friends. He published his *Materia Medica Pura* in 1810, and included 67 remedies (*see* Chapter Three).

In 1810 Hahnemann published *The Organon of the Rational Art of Healing* in which he defined his ideas and which, before his death, had attained its fifth edition. It was translated into several languages and in 1833 it appeared in English; three years later it was published in America.

The following are just two extracts:

> The highest ideal of cure is speedy, gentle and enduring restoration to health . . .

and

> The human body is, in its living state, a unity, a complete and rounded whole. Every sensation, every manifestation of force, every inter-relation of the material of one part, is intimately concerned with the sensation, force manifestations and inter-relations of all the other parts . . .

Twice Hahnemann was able to put his findings to the test.

In 1812, in the severest winter weather, Napoleon's army were starving whilst wending their way homewards across

Europe. The aftermath was a terrible epidemic of typhoid. Hahnemann treated 180 cases – only one died. From this point his fame spread throughout Europe.

In 1831 cholera swept towards western Europe. Hahnemann at once set about finding a cure and proved at the outset that camphor was the most likely. He wrote and printed several pamphlets, but his enemies were doing everything possible to prevent the spread of his teachings. Surprisingly, however, his suggestions did spread from one country to another and good results were reported from all quarters where his ideas were practised.

During the cholera epidemic the British doctor F. F. Quin, who had already met Hahnemann on one occasion, travelled to Moravia in order to study the disease and investigate more deeply the homoeopathic treatment. On his return to London, a convinced homoeopath now, he set up practice in St James's. In 1844, with help from friends, he founded The London Homoeopathic Hospital (now The Royal London Homoeopathic Hospital) and in this way homoeopathy became established in Britain.

Soon after Hahnemann's 75th birthday his wife died. Five years later he married Melanie d'Hervilly, a woman half his age. In 1835 they moved to Paris where Hahnemann was consulted by doctors and scientists from far and wide. He died in 1843.

CHAPTER 2

The Vital Force

In order to explain how homoeopathy differs from allopathic medicine it is necessary to expand on what I have called the vital force. Hahnemann believed that disease and its cure by homoeopathic remedies could only be explained by the acceptance of a vital principle (vital force) animating the body, and a similar vital principle or force embodied in every medicinal substance. Among the first paragraphs of the *Organon* Hahnemann explains the broad dividing line between the homoeopathic system of medicine and the old school in his recognition of the dynamic vitality or life force of the organism. He tells us that it is in this life power, this invisible principle, that we should look for the disturbing agent in sickness. It is dynamic, not material. It is this power or vital force which, when we are healthy, protects us against all disease. Susceptibility to the elements, to disease-producing agents, depends upon a lowered vitality or weakened dynamic or life force. Hahnemann says it is the first and highest duty of the physician to employ such means as will increase the strength of this dynamic resisting power and restore health.

This places the system of Hahnemann upon a different basis from that of orthodox medicine. The homoeopath is dealing with the dynamic effects of deranged vitality (which we call disease). Physicians of the other school may be dealing with the same thing, but they attempt to control vital derangement by mechanical or material means.

The life force, the vital force, is the force without which man ceases to be in his accustomed form, the force which operates and controls the operations of physical man and the organs of which he is composed; the force which makes it possible for the physical man to exist as such – the animation, the life, the controlling force, the spirit. It is the dynamism that animates and rules the body, retaining all the parts of the organism in harmonious, vital operation, as regards both sensations and function. It is the force which governs waste and repair. It is the builder of tissues. So long as that force is operating undisturbed, every organ, every tissue and cell is functioning in perfect harmony, and a state of absolute health prevails. Man is unconscious of his organs and their operations so long as perfect equilibrium is maintained, but once that equilibrium is disturbed the harmonious operation ceases to exist.

Manifestations of disturbances are evidenced in nature's own language – symptoms. Man becomes conscious of these and says, 'I feel unwell'. His sensations and functions are disturbed and later cell changes and pathological conditions come to light.

It is very important to understand that the vital force is attacked first, and as it flows through every part of the body, even to the minutest cell, we must look upon the patient as a complete unit, different from any other human being; every man is unique and a little world in himself. Certainly we have to take note of signs and symptoms – this is the only way we have of ascertaining the presence of disease – but it is the vital force which must be put right, harmonized, returned to a state of equilibrium, before cure can be effected.

To remove symptoms is not always the same thing as to cure. Unhappily, most sick people today are only interested in the removal of symptoms, and this can be done very effectively by palliation. But do you not see that by palliating symptoms nothing is done to help the vital force to return to normality, and that the state of sickness still pervades the system? It has tried to make its presence felt by signs and symptoms in order that it might be cured, but now the situation is worse because the vital force is still out of harmony and more damage is being inflicted on the physical body.

If, on the other hand, when these signs and symptoms first appear, homoeopathic treatment is used, then inquiries are made about the patient as a whole and how he differs from his healthy norm, in addition to the symptoms of the physical manifestation.

The vital force is present in every living substance (otherwise the substance would be inert), and when homoeopathic medicines are prescribed for sick patients, they too contain the life force (vital force) which we are discussing. The remedy needed by the patient is that which matches his 'totality of symptoms'; then his vital force is stimulated and returned to harmony. When that happens the patient will say, 'I feel well' – some go further and say, 'I feel as though I have been integrated' – and one by one the signs and symptoms disappear; there is nothing left to keep them in ultimation.

CHAPTER 3

Proving Homoeopathic Remedies

'By no effort of the mind can the curative properties of medicines be discovered in themselves.'

Organon

It was Hahnemann who decided that the only way to learn about homoeopathic remedies and what they can cure is to test them on healthy human beings. Symptoms of the mind are very important in this context as they form an integral part of the whole patient – they must be cured as well as physical symptoms, and it is essential that the reactions of the remedies in relation to the mind and emotions are known. And so Hahnemann enlisted the help of his family and friends in the task of proving the first medicines. Small doses of a substance were administered to all taking part in the proving, but the subjects were not told what they were given. All were in possession of notebooks and were asked to write down everything they felt and noticed.

These provings became more and more interesting to Hahnemann because he soon realized that many provers (but not all) were experiencing similar symptoms. As the days went by more and more symptoms developed, some peculiar to men, some to women, and many peculiar to both. Nearly all the provers developed some symptoms, about half developed others, and only a very few provers developed the remaining symptoms. I mention this because the symptoms brought out by nearly all the provers are strongly characteristic of that medicine and are printed in thick black type in the homoeopathic repertories; symptoms in the next category are printed in italic, and those registered by only a very few provers are in ordinary type. This allows the prescriber to see at a glance if the medicine and the patient both show strongly marked symptoms.

Apart from very high fevers, terrible nausea and vomiting, ghastly aches and pains in the limbs, and difficult breathing, to name only a very few symptoms, deep depression, thoughts of suicide, emotional stress with bouts of weeping, anger, great fears, anxieties, and lack of concentration all came to light. We have only to read some of the provings to realize perhaps a little of what the provers suffered. For instance, under *Aurum Metallicum* (Gold) we read:

Feeling of self-condemnation and utter worthlessness. Profound despondency, with increased blood-pressure, with thorough disgust of life, and thoughts of suicide. Talks of committing suicide. Great fear of death. Peevish and vehement at least contradiction. Mental derangements. Constant rapid questioning without waiting for reply. Cannot do things fast enough. Over-sensitiveness to noise, excitement and confusion.

And under *Belladonna* (Deadly Nightshade) we find:

Patient lives in a world of his own, engrossed by spectres and visions and oblivious to surrounding realities. While the retina is insensible to actual objects, a host of visual hallucinations throng about him and come to him from within. He is acutely alive, crazed by a flood of subjective visual impressions and fantastic illusions. Hallucinations, sees monsters, hideous faces; delirium; frightful images; furious; rages, bites, strikes, desire to escape. Loss of consciousness. Disinclined to talk. Perversity with tears. Acuteness of all senses. Changeableness.

We go on to *Hyoscyamus* (Henbane) and read:

Very suspicious. Talkative; obscene; lascivious mania; uncovers body; jealous; foolish. Great hilarity; inclined to laugh at everything. Delirium with attempt to run away. Low muttering speech; deep stupor.

I cannot leave out *Lachesis* (Poison from the Surucucuo snake). Dr Constantine Hering, who was a pupil of Hahnemann, compiled ten volumes of *materia medica* called *Hering's Guiding Symptoms*; these included the provings of *Lachesis* which occupied almost one hundred pages! Dr J. H. Clarke, in his *Dictionary of Materia Medica*, states under Lachesis:

To the genius and the heroism of Hering the world owes this remedy and many another of which this has been the forerunner. When Hering's first experiments were made he was botanizing and zoologizing on the upper Amazon for the German Government. Except his wife, all those around him were natives who told him so much about the dreaded Surukuku that he offered a good reward for a live specimen. At last one was brought in a bamboo box and those who brought it immediately fled, and all his native servants with them.

Hering stunned the snake with a blow on the head as the box opened, then holding its head in a forked stick, he pressed its venom out of the poison bag upon sugar of milk. The effect of handling the virus and preparing the lower attenuations was to throw Hering into a fever, with tossing delirium and mania – much to his wife's dismay. Towards morning he slept and on waking his mind was clear. He drank a little water to moisten his throat and the first question this indomitable prover asked was, 'What did I do and say?' His wife remembered vividly enough. The symptoms were written down and his was the first instalment of *Lachesis*.

Subsequently it was fully proved. Some of the mental symptoms are:

Great loquacity. Amative. Sad in the morning, no desire to mix with the world. Restless and uneasy; does not wish to attend to business. Wants to be off somewhere all the time. Jealous. Mental labour best performed at night. Euthanasia. Suspicious; nightly delusion of fire. Religious insanity. Derangement of the time sense.

Natrum muriaticum (Chloride of Sodium, common salt) is interesting:

Psychic causes of disease; ill effects of grief, fright, anger, etc. Depressed; particularly in chronic disease. Consolation aggravates. Irritable, gets into a passion about trifles. Awkward hasty. Wants to be alone to weep. Tears with laughter.

And lastly *Stramonium* (Thorn-apple):

Devout, earnest, beseeching and ceaseless talking. Loquacious, garrulous, laughing, singing, swearing, praying, rhyming. Sees ghosts, hears voices, talks with spirits. Rapid changes from joy to sadness. Violent and lewd. Delusions about his identity; thinks himself tall, double, a part missing. Religious mania. Cannot bear solitude or darkness; must have light and company. Sight of water or anything glistening brings on spasms.

These extracts are taken from Boericke's *Homoeopathic Materia Medica* to give an insight as to the kind of symptoms that can be treated in mentally sick patients. When a substance is fully proven all the symptoms are sorted under various headings. And so it is that the prescriber can look up the indicated remedy in a number of excellent works; all the information known is available.

At the time of his death, Hahnemann had sixty proven remedies; today there are at least 2000. The homoeopath has, indeed, a good armoury.

CHAPTER 4

Potentization

When Hahnemann found that large doses of the indicated remedy made the condition worse he began experiments to reduce dosage to the minimum quantity sufficient to cure the sickness. In addition to being a doctor he was also an analytical chemist, and so his task was not too difficult. Finally he found the answer. To one drop of the mother tincture (or any soluble substance) he added ninety-nine drops of diluent, usually distilled water; this was shaken to make the 1st centesimal potency. One drop of this potency was added to ninety-nine drops of diluent and shaken well, making the 2nd centesimal potency. One drop of the 2nd potency was added to ninety-nine drops of diluent and shaken well, making the 3rd potency, and so on until the 30th potency was attained. This can be expressed as a fraction of one over one followed by sixty noughts!

Later, followers of Hahnemann potentized remedies to a much higher degree, the most used being the 6th, 12th, 30th, 200th, 1000th (1M) and the 10m. Sometimes the CM and the MM are required, but not very often.

If the substance to be potentized is insoluble in water then one part is added to ninety-nine parts of sugar of milk and triturated in a pestle and mortar, making the 1st centesimal trituration. One part of this is mixed with ninety-nine parts of sugar of milk and triturated, making the 2nd trituration. When the 4th trituration has been attained the substance becomes soluble and the procedure is as above until the required potency is obtained.

Constantine Hering, a pupil of Hahnemann, introduced the decimal system of potentization. One drop of the mother tincture is added to nine drops of diluent and shaken well to make the 1st decimal potency. One drop of this is added to nine drops of diluent and shaken well to make the 2nd decimal potency, and so on until the required potency is reached. Again, if an insoluble substance is used then one part is added to nine parts of sugar of milk and triturated in a pestle and mortar to make the 1st decimal trituration. This is continued until the 7th trituration has been attained when the substance becomes soluble; subsequently, potentization is continued by adding one drop to nine of diluent.

The centesimal scale may be marked with a 'c' or 'CH' (Continental), e.g. *Arnica* 6c, but generally the 'c' is omitted and whenever a number follows the name of the remedy, e.g. *Arnica* 6, the centesimal scale is understood. An 'x' always follows the number of the potency in the decimal scale.

Each time a remedy is potentized, more of the physical substance is removed, and by the time the 30th potency is reached analysis shows no trace of it. But also during potentization the 'energy' or 'power' of the substance is released, the specific energy required by the body for healing, the energy that restores the vital force to harmony, thus making the patient whole – integrated. As the process continues to the higher potencies, so that energy becomes greater, more powerful. This must be difficult to understand when first confronted with these facts, but it is something that the homoeopath is proving every day. One of the laws of prescribing is 'Never change the remedy whilst the patient is improving'; so having found the medicine to fit the patient's symptoms this medicine is prescribed in the most suitable potency. I often begin to treat a case of chronic disease with the 30th. The patient may improve quite considerably and then there may be a period when nothing very much happens. The same remedy in the same potency is repeated. Still there is no further improvement. Then the same remedy in a higher potency (the 200th) is given, and the patient improves greatly – and is often cured. The 30th potency takes the patient a little way along the path and then can do no more – but the greater energy in the 200th continues the curing process and if necessary the thousandth and even higher potencies can be used. If the symptoms alter the remedy has to be changed, and then the same rules apply again.

An interesting aspect of homoeopathic remedies is that they will keep almost indefinitely providing they are stored correctly. This should not be difficult to understand if we think of each medicine in terms of energy or power and *not* as a material substance. But they *are* sensitive – to bright sunlight and to odours (perfumes, soaps, cigarette smoke, etc.). They should therefore be kept in a drawer or cupboard away from any of the above, preferably in glass containers with tight-fitting caps. Then they will still work and be effective in twenty to thirty years' time! Remedies should never be transferred to a bottle that has contained a different medicine or the same medicine in a different potency.

All homoeopathic medicines should be prepared by a chemist specializing in this type of pharmacy.

CHAPTER 5

The Laws of Cure

We have many guidelines in homoeopathy. Curative action occurs in three ways and is marked by the development of symptoms:

1. From centre to circumference.
2. From above down.
3. In the reverse order of appearance.

Let us consider these three laws.

1. *From the centre to the circumference.* Crises of elimination often occur as a skin eruption, bouts of diarrhoea, an increased flow of urine, a fever with much sweating, or symptoms of a very bad cold. Thus the poisons are being driven out of the body from the centre.

2. *From above down.* If rheumatic pains are suffered in the arms or shoulders they may travel to the hands and fingers; if there are pains in the hips they may go down to the feet before they are eliminated.

3. *Symptoms disappear in the reverse order of their appearance.* If a patient comes for treatment with a skin eruption but says she used to suffer with severe headaches, then during the course of treatment the skin may clear and the headaches may return. These clear up and then the patient is cured – the third law has been illustrated. As another example, in measles the cough comes first and departs last, the rash arrives last and goes first. In cases of chronic disease it has been proved over and over again that the patient will retrace the road along which the disease has travelled and in so doing he will experience again the various ailments from which he has suffered in the past, until he returns to the condition in which his troubles began. When this is eradicated he is cured. In many cases this is a long and difficult

process – rather than a straight road to cure the process manifests itself as a spiral, although eventually the upward trend predominates and the reversals are less frequent and of shorter duration.

The prescriber must never interfere with the action of a remedy by giving another too quickly. When there is an aggravation and old symptoms reappear, the patient always begs for quick relief; nothing must be prescribed at this stage (except unmedicated pills as a placebo) because these symptoms are being brought to the surface for elimination. This is very important and must be understood at the outset.

These laws are applicable in all forms of disease and are the criteria by which the practitioner judges the progress of the patient. When the most similar remedy is administered the practitioner must wait for results. It may be that in a few days other symptoms will appear. If this reaction is in the form of an eruption on the skin, diarrhoea, or a sneezing cold, as I mentioned earlier poisons are being eradicated from the centre of the patient and brought to the surface and all is going well. The rhythm of the remedy must not be interfered with by administering another at this point. Gradually, the aggravation will subside and then the patient will usually say, 'I feel so much better in myself', even though his aches and pains are still with him. But when the 'I' feels better then we know that we are working from the innermost of the economy.

It may take a long time to cure a chronic disorder; many things have to be taken into consideration and this is no easy task. From time to time the remedy has to be repeated or altered according to the symptoms, and these must be watched closely. But, throughout, the homoeopath has guidelines – he knows what should be prescribed and from the symptoms he can assess whether the patient is on the right road. He does not have to experiment; he does not have to worry about side effects. Homoeopathy works with and within the laws of nature, and in so doing the patient is integrated and made whole.

CHAPTER 6

The Miasms

1. PSORA

Knowledge of the miasms is absolutely essential to the successful practice of homoeopathy. So many of us start at the wrong end without this knowledge and spend many years doing mediocre work and feeling frustrated as we are without a valuable key which can undo some very stubborn locks. Very often the similimum is selected and given in the correct potency, and yet cure does not come to the patient. This can be puzzling and disappointing, but it brings me to the crux of the matter. There is a state in the organism which blocks the way to the apparently indicated remedy, and to this state Hahnemann gave the name 'miasm'. It is to the genius of Hahnemann, to his prodigious research, to his endless patience and indomitable courage, that we owe our gratitude for this priceless knowledge. He was led to research along these lines by his observation of the fact that there were states in some patients which simply did not yield to the similar remedy. He observed that there was nothing in external causes such as diet or mode of life to account for this state. So Hahnemann allotted himself twelve years to research into and meditate upon this question. During these twelve years he did not speak or write about the problem. His research took the form of inquiry into hundreds of case histories where he laboriously traced back into the patients' inheritance as far as was possible. He traced back into the ancient origin of primal disease in the history of all nations, even, we are told, into the ancient Oriental. After endless difficulties he traced the origin of disease to what was called the 'Itch' disease, an eruption upon the skin. To this condition he gave the name Psora. The derivation of the word

Psora is either Latin or Greek, but it is suggested that it is further derived from the Hebrew word 'Tsorat', meaning a fault, a groove, a pollution or a stigma, such as would apply to the leprous manifestations and the great plagues of those times. In modern language we should name this term 'constitutional defect'.

What in essence is Psora? The itching eruption is not Psora but merely its manifestation. Psora itself is a condition of the system which enables it to develop disease. So Psora itself is invisible; all that are visible are its effects, which are innumerable. Almost all skin diseases, other than the eruptions of venereal diseases, are Psoric. All itching, whether with or without eruption, is Psoric. It is the base from which leprosy sprang, and is also the base from which all eruptive diseases of the Earth originated. Hahnemann refers us to the third book of Moses where Psora is described.

The miasm of Psora has, through the centuries, polluted the human bloodstream through hereditary transmissions, but in the course of transmission it has been much modified. It is seen less in its primary manifestation as skin disease but is now the invisible incubus from which a whole host of other symptoms spring. Hahnemann declared Psora to be the mother of all disease and claimed that without its presence in the human organism the other miasms of Syphilis and Gonorrhoea could not implant themselves. He also suggested that in earlier times, when Psora manifested itself upon the skin, the internal organism was greatly relieved and people enjoyed a greater sense of well-being, but that its suppression by such means as the application of ointments, the use of X-rays, etc., has forced it inwards where it causes a great deal of functional disturbance. Every practitioner can from his own experience verify the fact that when an eruption is thrown out upon the skin the internal organs are generally relieved and the patient feels better in himself.

How may we recognize Psora in the human organism?

The first thing we note is that its operations are mainly functional, that it never produces structural changes. When those are present we must look for Syphilis or Sycosis in the system. The Psoric patient is nervous and restless and full of anxiety, depression, fears and sensations, and suffers from much palpitation and heart fluttering. When this develops he is always convinced that his end is near and he will sit in quiet fixedness awaiting it. The Psoric patient is sensitive in mind and body. He has an abundance of ideas and his mind moves so fast that he mentally trips over himself. He is often of a philosophical turn of mind and is interested in the whys and wherefores of the universe. He is often subject to flashes of inventive genius but is never stable enough to achieve anything or to come to any conclusion. He jumps from one thing to another, starting many things and finishing nothing. In the physical sphere this restlessness is also expressed. The Psoric patient is quick in body movements and works very hard but gets tired quickly and wants to lie down. That is another strong characteristic of Psora; the necessity to lie down and the feeling of relief when doing so. Psora, in fact, affects every function and has numerous stomach and bowel symptoms. The patient is always hungry, craving innumerable and unsuitable foods. He craves sweet things and sour things and feels weak and hungry at 11 o'clock in the morning. Headaches, always severe, are brought on by emotion, looking up, and rising. They come on with the rising of the sun and get better with its setting, and are often accompanied by a flushed face and pulsations. The patient's hair is harsh and dry and often falls out after illness. It becomes grey early in life and often produces white spots or streaks. The scalp is dry with scaly eruptions which itch considerably. There are no structural changes in the eye but the patient often suffers spots before the vision and he finds strong sunlight very trying. Ears again show no structural change but they are sensitive and such patients suffer severely if exposed to noise. The face is often dry, hot and shining with dry, harsh skin, very red lips, red ears, red-rimmed eyes. The face often has a triangular appearance. In his colds and chest troubles, of which he has many, the Psoric patient is always greatly alarmed and regards the affection as serious when it is not so. But over-sensitivity, both mental and physical, is truly characteristic of the Psoric patient, who is sooner brought low by grief and unhappiness than by any physical hardship.

Another peculiarity of the Psoric patient is that he thoroughly dislikes washing and bathing; he quite happily endures dirty shirts and frayed cuffs, and is generally indifferent to his appearance. For this state *Sulphur* is the classic remedy, although it is not suitable for treating all cases of Psora. Fifty-three other remedies are listed for this state and, of course, *Psorinum*, the product of scabies, is a close runner-up and is often needed if *Sulphur*, although indicated, fails.

Dr Roberts, in his book *The Principles and Art of Cure by Homoeopathy*, argues the case that Psora and deficiency are interchangeable terms. He brings to our notice the interesting fact that nearly all Psoric remedies are the same weight as the elements of body construction. It has been established that when the diet lacks, or the body fails to assimilate, any of these body elements (sodium, calcium, oxygen, etc.), disturbance in health occurs. An experimental diet was given to certain animals from which various minerals were excluded, and it was proved that grave derangement in their emotional and physical organism occurred; this was corrected when the missing elements were replaced in the diet in the infinitesimal quantities that nature requires. Psora in the system is responsible for the imperfect assimilation of elements necessary for perfect body functioning and resultant deficiencies, whether of air, food, sunlight or rest. Hahnemann named Psora the mother of all disease and declared that without its presence in the system the other two great miasms, Syphilis and Gonorrhoea, could not have obtained a stranglehold. Only the presence of Psora made the organism receptive to their influence.

2. SYPHILIS

The second miasm, Syphilis, becomes from the first moment of infection a constitutional disease. The incubation period is three weeks. In that short time, and in a silent, imperceptible and thorough way, the disease insinuates itself completely into the organism. The life force meets the crisis by throwing it out upon the surface of the body in the form of a chancre and the inner man is thereby relieved. But nature is ignored by man who makes every effort to dry the chancre up and in this way returns the poison to the internal system. The vital force then makes a second attempt to cast the disease off by means of a skin eruption, and here again orthodox medical treatment thwarts nature's safeguard by suppressing the eruption with ointments and damming up the outlet. The infection now vents all its venom upon the nervous system, the blood vessels and the heart. By virtue of perseverance of the same policy, this new derangement is further suppressed, resulting in ulcerations of skin, bones, liver and large blood vessels. In this stage the miasm has seized the organism in a stranglehold which is not released until death claims the victim.

This blight is perpetuated in any offspring, but does not now manifest itself in the first stage of ulcer or chancre for by this time it has become so united with the life force as to be inseparable and now shows itself through chronic catarrhal states, bone deformities, liver affections and anaemia. The brain shares in this blight with resultant slowness of thought and poor memory.

Syphilitics are often very difficult to live with for they are depressed, sullen, self-reproachful and often 'pig-headed'. Their stubbornness is their defence mechanism against livelier personalities and the fast-moving current of life which they find themselves unable to cope with. A knowledge of this basic taint helps us to be patient when dealing with them. One of the hallmarks of the syphilitic condition is time aggravation. Patients are always worse at night; indeed, their symptoms, especially restlessness, are so much worse at night that they fear its onset and the consequent great exhaustion they feel on waking. Outward manifestations such as ulcers and discharges of leucorrhoea and catarrh relieve the mental condition and the internal organs. Headaches caused by this miasm can be recognized by their coming on at night and the fact that they have their point of departure at the base of the brain. They are aggravated or brought on by mental or physical effort, and children tainted with this miasm often, in their illness, bore their heads into the pillow. The giddiness of blood-pressure caused by thickening of the arteries is one of the structural changes caused by syphilis.

Congenital syphilis can be recognized in the appearance of the head, which is large and unshapely with hair that is sticky and greasy. Patients often complain of pains in the skull. This miasm does not favour the growth of hair and often growth is perverted, for eyelashes and beard sometimes grow inward. Frequently, hair and eyebrows fall out. Moist and scabby eruptions appear on the scalp, which often perspires profusely. In the nose there is destruction of tissue and sometimes even the bones are destroyed, especially the bridge of the nose. A flattened bridge tells us to look for the presence of this miasm in the patient. Scabs and crusts which bleed when removed as well as haemorrhage and loss of smell are also pointers to this taint. In the mouth there is much ulceration and structural defects exemplified by the irregularity of the teeth and their decay; the dental arch is often deformed.

The syphilitic is extremely sensitive to weather changes. He catches cold very easily and frequently suffers from enlarged tonsils and adenoids. This state of affairs is bad enough but the position is far worse when the Psoric miasm unites with the syphilitic; the offspring of this ill-fated union is tuberculosis. Perhaps a word about the tubercular state as distinct from straight-forward tuberculosis might be appropriate here. The victims of this miasm are always 'dead-tired' and always seek the recumbent position; they are better in the daytime and worse at night, showing here the influence of the syphilitic miasm. They have narrow chests and as a result poor chest expansion limits the intake of oxygen, causing anaemia. This in its turn maims the digestive system, resulting in poor nutrition, and in this way a vicious circle is set up. The tubercular miasm is the hidden enemy behind such troubles as diabetes, hernia, varicose veins and some heart troubles.

Miasms yield to treatment. Knowledge and experience are needed to treat these states – bungling and inexperience can cause suppression in which the final condition is worse than the first; the responsibility of the prescriber is great.

3. SYCOSIS

Sycosis, the third miasm, is the result of suppressed gonorrhoea. We all know that after infection by the gonococci acute inflammation of the genital tract occurs some five to ten days later. This state can be met and cured by homoeopathy, but unfortunately most sufferers seek allopathic treatment which succeeds only in driving inwards the manifestations of the inflammation, producing a latent state of illness to which the name Sycosis is given. Frustrated in its attempt to push out to the surface, the disease vents its energy upon the internal organs and succeeds in vitiating the blood-stream, resulting in a state of anaemia. This gives rise to a vicious circle of catarrhal infections and an inflammatory condition of the internal tissues which manifests itself in rheumatism. The victim seeking relief from this further disaster is again met by unscientific methods of alleviation which further suppress the malady and chase the disorder into the depths of the mind and nervous system.

In this condition the sufferer is beyond all human aid.

The repercussions of Sycosis are endless once the process is set in motion. We observe it in cases where the so-called 'cured' husband passes it on to his unsuspecting wife. Before marriage she was full of abounding health and vitality but shortly afterwards she begins to 'dwindle and pine' as a result of the transmission of secondary Sycosis. This announces its establishment in the organism by inflammation of the ovaries and fallopian tubes, and by the presence of severe anaemia due to the power of Sycosis to destroy the red corpuscles. These conditions are pointers to possible future malignancy if not corrected by the similar remedy before a complete stranglehold has been obtained.

The mind and nervous system are spheres where Sycosis wreaks serious damage, creating abnormal states of jealousy, suspicion, loss of memory and violent temper. Sycosis, when united with Psora, creates mental degeneracy resulting in suicidal tendencies, criminality and insanity. External manifestations such as warts, catarrhal discharges, leucorrhoea, growths and ulcerations greatly relieve the mental state when they appear.

Sycosis, unlike Psora which is responsible for functional changes only, is the force which produces structural changes exemplified by stunted growths of hair and falling of hair from head and beard. It is also the power behind rheumatism and the deformities of arthritis. It is seen again in the proliferation of tissue evinced in warts, thickened skin, callosities, thickened nails and all kinds of tumours and growths. When tumours are malignant we may look for the presence of the Syphilitic and Psoric miasms in combination with Sycosis.

Those of us who practise homoeopathy have the task of unravelling these miasms with the appropriate remedies and treating each as it predominates. In this way some tangles can be straightened out and the organism freed of the miasms. But this is not always possible. Sometimes it is too difficult to unravel the knot that has been tied, particularly if many crude drugs have been taken along the road. However, in a great percentage of these cases good results are obtained after much patience and study, thanks to the teaching and guidance of Samuel Hahnemann.

CHAPTER 7

Vaccinosis

A brilliant homoeopathic physician, Dr James Compton Burnett (*see* Chapter Seventeen), wrote an extremely interesting little book towards the end of the 19th century called *Vaccinosis*, a term coined by him. By this he means the disease which results from vaccination, plus 'that profound and often long-lasting morbid constitutional state engendered by the vaccine virus'. He questions the term 'lymph' (the substance used in vaccination) and suggests that in reality this is nothing but 'pus' or matter. And when we think of pus being induced into our blood-streams it certainly gives rise to thought. In many cases people are healthy when they are vaccinated in order, for example, that they do not catch smallpox. So when a *diseased* state has been introduced, this then makes them immune? Dr Burnett states that those people who 'do not take' – in other words those who do not suffer any aggravations at the time of the vaccination are in a worse position than those whose built-in defence mechanism fights the poison with resultant suppuration. In these cases the pus enters the economy, usually to cause trouble later.

Many patients of mine have said when questioned closely (because the cause of their trouble has not been apparent), 'I haven't been really well since I was vaccinated.' A statement like this supplies the missing link in an otherwise baffling case. No constitutional remedy will restore harmony if vaccinal poison blocks the way.

We have in our *materia medica Thuja Occidentalis* (*Arbor vitae* or the Tree of Life). This remedy was a discovery of Hahnemann, and practically nothing was known of its properties until he proved it. Dr Clarke tells us, 'Hahnemann found in *Thuja* the antidote to the miasm of the condition he called Sycosis.' Boenninghausen, a pupil of Hahnemann, found *Thuja* both preventive and curative in an epidemic of smallpox. Following this, Drs Kinkel and Goullon proved this same remedy to be curative of the ill-effects of vaccination, or as Dr Burnett calls it, Vaccinosis – the symptoms are similar.

Dr J. A. Allen states in his work *The Chronic Miasms*, 'I wish to say a few words about another mode of entrance of the sycotic poison into the organism, and that is through the vicious method of vaccination, now in vogue. We believe this to be a form of sycosis, indeed we have no longer a doubt about it . . . vaccination causes all races to be sycotic and is the father of a multitude of skin diseases such as erysipelas, impetigo, psoriasis, morbelliform rashes, some forms of gangrene, erythemas, roseola, papular and pustular eruptions of different forms, urticaria, eczema, dermatitis, herpetiformis, pemphigus of one form, lupus vulgaris and many others that may be mentioned. All cry out, "Stop the death-dealing process of vaccination or the whole race will soon become degenerate." '

Orthodox doctors admit nothing of all this, and so patients who consult them when not feeling well from vaccinal poison arc probably prescribed drugs that will suppress their symptoms and aggravate the condition, not only for them but for future generations. Today most people are vaccinated without second thought. If they travel abroad, vaccination every three years is compulsory when going to countries like South Africa and America.

Until this part of the Sycotic miasm is recognized and treated homoeopathically – in other words removed from the system – the sickness of man will become an even larger Gordian knot which, in some cases, will become impossible to unravel.

CHAPTER 8

Taking the Case

To make whole is to cure, and if one is to cure the patient a great deal of information must be obtained, not only about the complaint from which he is suffering, but about the man himself and how that sickness has made him *different from his norm.* For he is a little world in himself, different from anybody else.

When a patient presents himself for treatment of some chronic disease the first thing the practitioner must do is to listen to all he has to say about his troubles, the sickness that he has come to have cured. The fullest notes must be taken and, when he has finished, details must be filled in by questions from the prescriber. What makes your aches and pains better (heat, cold, pressure, and so on)? Is there any time in the twenty-four hours when they are better – or worse? The type of pain must be clarified – is it burning, sore, stitching ... Describe the pain in your own words. Describe your cough in your own words, and if there is mucus details of this must be given also. When all the details of the actual illness have been covered, then we turn to previous and family history. The patient is asked to give details of all the troubles he has had from childhood, and any really serious illnesses should be underlined for reference later. Details of family history must be taken, any serious illness of parents, grand-parents, sisters, brothers, and near relatives.

Now we turn to the man himself, and I always begin by asking, In what weather do you feel happiest? Answers always give a clue as to whether the symptom is marked or not. Hesitation or a response such as 'Well, I don't think ...' means that we can forget the answers because they are of no value. Those that help to put the jigsaw together are spontaneous and come forth with clarity and force . . . 'I cannot do anything in the heat, it makes me feel really ill, especially since my . . . started' – this is a marked symptom and must be taken into consideration when prescribing.

From weather to food. Are there any foods which you cannot eat? What about fats, sweets, salt? Do you enjoy your food? What would happen if you had to miss a meal? How do you feel in-between meals, especially mid-morning? Give me an example of typical meals for a day. Do you cook in aluminium pots and pans? How much and what do you drink during the course of the day? Full information must be obtained regarding bowels, bladder, perspiration and, if applicable, menses. What about sleep – full details must be given. How many times has the patient been vaccinated against smallpox?

Having secured the confidence of the patient, now is the time to ask about the 'essential' man. What about anger, irritability, impatience? Describe any fears or anxieties. Do you get het up anticipating events? When sick or in trouble, do you like being fussed and consoled? Do you weep easily? Are you a sensitive person, and if so to what? How do you react to heights, to crowds, and closed-in spaces? What about concentration and capacity for thinking?

These are general questions covering the majority of cases, but no doubt I shall be told that some have been omitted. As the consultation progresses, questions come to mind peculiar to a particular patient, for example, questions pertaining to his or her sex-life or, if the patient is very unbalanced, any thoughts of suicide and so on. I have learned over the years that a practitioner must have a very 'elastic' approach which must be adapted to each patient.

Everything that is marked in the patient and in his sickness must be underlined, because these symptoms must be strongly marked in the constitutional remedy also.

This book has not been written for teaching purposes but to give the 'man in the street' an insight into the nature of homoeopathy, how it differs from orthodox medicine, and how the patient is treated. It is not necessary to discuss the method of finding the correct remedy, but suffice it to say that unless the full facts of the case are known it is doubtful whether the remedy that is similar to the sickness will be found. I always make it quite clear to my patients that this is a two-way effort. They must first of all help by giving a clear picture of their sickness and of themselves, and subsequently they must give accurate progress reports.

It is usual for a patient to receive treatment for one month – full instructions are given and at the same time they are requested to make notes of anything they feel or notice during the four weeks – otherwise it is impossible to remember what has happened and the correct sequence of events. It is by comparing one month with another that we can see the trend of the patient's progress. I encourage patients to contact me during the month if at any time they feel worried or have any queries, and in this way I usually win co-operation and trust. Patients are grateful that I spend an hour over the first consultation – no homoeopath can do otherwise, and the fact that they are encouraged to talk and go into the details of their problems relieves pent-up emotions.

CHAPTER 9

Past History of the Patient

If the correct homoeopathic prescription is to be made the case history of the patient must be taken very carefully. After assessing the symptoms of the patient as a whole, together with those of the trouble for which he has come to be cured, a remedy is prescribed. The similimum may be easy to find; alternatively, some cases need a great deal of thought and study. Many cases bring satisfactory results from the beginning – others are just as difficult!

It is in such situations that we often find the answer in the past history of the patient. The constitutional remedy will work more often than not, but failure to achieve results means that we have to look further into the case for some clue that may give us the key, unless, of course, the wrong prescription was given in the first place! We may find that the patient has suffered from an acute infection during the previous weeks or months which has lowered vitality. Homoeopathic remedies such as *Sulphur* or *Psorium* will often eradicate the trouble and the patient may not need anything else. The remedy must be carefully selected according to the infection. The childish ailments can sometimes cause illness in later life, even in adulthood. It is always wise to underline, for instance 'I had measles *very* badly as a child', and if this is a factor then *Morbillinum* will clear up the trouble or make way for the constitutional medicine to do so. If the vital force is unable to annihilate the poison from measles it can lie dormant in the system until something brings it to life again. 'I have never been well since . . .' should alert the prescriber to the possibility that a nosode may be necessary, but providing there are good indications for the constitutional remedy this should always be prescribed first.

The after-effects of vaccination, immediate or remote, can play havoc in some constitutions. I have cleared up many cases that did not respond to the constitutional medicine by giving *Thuja* on the evidence of several vaccinations. Symptoms created by the smallpox vaccination are similar to those of the sycotic miasm, and *Thuja* is a great sycotic remedy.

If injuries are not dealt with satisfactorily they can cause suffering subsequently. A patient came to see me not long ago suffering from pains in her arm and hand. There was not very much on which to prescribe until she remembered she had fallen in her garden about six months previously. She had no immediate trouble after the bruising had gone, but gradually her arm and then her hand developed pains. I gave her nine doses of *Arnica* 30 and in one week all traces of the symptoms had disappeared. *Arnica* should always be remembered for injuries or for symptoms resulting from an injury – however remote (*see* Chapter Eleven).

Spinal injuries can cause havoc subsequently and sometimes symptoms seemingly quite unrelated can develop. Then *Hypericum* will ease the way and the patient will be cured of all troubles. I remember a young woman who came for relief from migraine headaches – she had at least one a week, and sometimes two, bad enough to make her retire to bed. The indicated remedy did very little, and after re-thinking the case, neither did the second medicine which was prescribed. What was in the background – what was stopping this patient from improving? After more careful questioning she revealed that she had fallen from some steps onto her 'tail' a few months previously, but did not think it was sufficiently important to mention, as after the initial pain and discomfort it had 'cleared up'. I gave her *Hypericum* and she had no migraine headaches for three and a half months, when they began to return but in a milder form. I repeated the *Hypericum* in higher potency and she had no more trouble.

I must also mention *Opium* which comes to mind for cases that will not clear up because of fright – but fright that can be recalled and relived even months or years afterwards. This sometimes applies to children who have been frightened when very young. Suddenly the fear will be recalled by some incident, and they will react by screaming or going very pale and quiet, or becoming ill. Adults too can relive a fright from years back which can cause physical symptoms such as asthma, skin troubles or headaches to manifest themselves. In these cases a dose of *Opium* will work wonders, for it will remove the cause of the disturbance.

Patients suffering from grief can derive great comfort from homoeopathy. They may have lost a loved one – husband, wife or close relative. Most people are naturally upset when such things happen, but gradually they pick up the threads of life again; they mix with people and adopt the motto 'life must go on'. But there are those who appear not to be able to make this effort, for effort it is, and they retire into their shells, rarely meeting people and becoming more and more depressed; here again physical symptoms often develop as an outcome. When they come for treatment it is often months or even a year or two after the event, and for these patients we turn to our 'grief' remedies – *Ignatia, Natrum muriaticum* or *Graphites* – according to their requirements.

And lastly, a brief mention of chloroform, because that too can cause trouble. Dr Donald Foubister, one-time paediatrician at The Royal London Homoeopathic Hospital, gave an interesting address to the Faculty of Homoeopathy on this subject. He said, 'For some years now I have taken "the anaesthetic history" of every patient, and this is occasionally very rewarding in constitutional prescribing. The most definite feature which has emerged is that patients suffering from liver or gall-bladder disease who have had a bad reaction to chloroform usually benefit from *Chloroform* in potency. A man of forty-five who had suffered from very severe attacks of asthma for ten years responded to some extent to constitutional treatment. He had been born under chloroform anaesthesia and his mother had been greatly upset by the anaesthetic. *Natrum sulph.* and *Lachesis*, both liver remedies, seemed to help him. He was given *Chloroform* 30 and later 200 and he has been practically free from asthma for over three years.' I myself had the case of a teenager who was suffering from frequent headaches with sickness. The indicated remedies did very little, and the mother informed me that the girl had been very upset by the anaesthetic when she had her tonsils and adenoids removed. Three doses of *Chloroform* completely wiped out the headaches and sickness.

There are many causes of disease, some more simple than others. But if a patient is to be cured, and the indicated constitutional remedy does not do all that is required, then the practitioner has to delve more deeply in a variety of ways, and past history often gives the answer. When the *full* facts of the case are known, it is then, and only then, that the correct remedy can be found.

CHAPTER 10

The Study of Homoeopathic Remedies

The study of homoeopathic remedies is quite different from that of crude drugs. We do not think in terms of which disease they will cure but concentrate on the symptoms which are marked in each one in order to match them with similar symptoms in the patient. Nobody can memorize the symptoms of all the remedies – indeed, it would be difficult to remember all the symptoms of one remedy. I have already said that there are about 2000 fully proven medicines in our *materia medicas* filling hundreds of pages.

But each remedy has a set of 'characteristic' symptoms; these have been suffered by *all* the provers, and they are the most important and are the main pointers for its use. The patient for whom the remedy has been prescribed does not need to exhibit all the characteristic symptoms, but if he has at least three which are strongly marked in his sickness then we can be assured that his physical symptoms will almost certainly show up in the provings and he will derive great benefit from the remedy.

The following six remedies are used constantly; all the symptoms given are characteristic of each one and are a key for prescribing.

Sulphur is the leading remedy and is known as 'the ragged philosopher'. (You will note from descriptions that we talk of our remedies as though they are people!) He is stoop-shouldered, lean and untidy; flings himself into a chair as standing is the most uncomfortable position for him. He is not very clean and children cannot bear to be washed. There is much burning, particularly of the feet, which are pushed out of bed at night. Skin itches which scratching relieves, followed by burning. Suffers weak, faint spells frequently throughout the day and has a weak all-gone feeling in the stomach mid-morning. All the orifices of the body are red – eyes, lips, nostrils and anus. Better fresh air.

I must make it clear that the above would be a classical *Sulphur* patient and if somebody with all the above symptoms presents himself for treatment then we are quite sure of our results. But, as I have said, the patient needing sulphur does not necessarily have all these symptoms and, indeed, he is rarely stoop-shouldered and dirty! Our minds must be very flexible when searching for the correct remedy.

Calcarea carbonica (Carbonate of Lime) is quite different from *Sulphur*. 'Fair, fat and flabby' are the words used in several *materia medicas* to describe this patient. Constitutionally fat or with a tendency to obesity, sluggish or slow in movement, always tired and weary, cold. Has a sensation in feet and legs as if she had on cold, damp stockings. Aversion to open air, the least cold goes right through her. Great debility, cannot walk far or go upstairs because of shortness of breath. Profuse sweating, especially on the heads of children at night, but the skin is cold. Body odour is sour. Easily strained from lifting.

Lycopodium (Club Moss) is different again. 'Thin, withered and full of gas' is one label attached to this remedy! This patient has great apprehension and fear when anticipating an unusual event, but is fine once he is actually participating. There is an aggravation of all symptoms between 4 and 8pm. Symptoms begin on the right side and often move across to the left. Has a full-up feeling after only a few mouthfuls of food. Extreme tendency to flatulence with intolerance of tight clothing.

Pulsatilla (Wind Flower) is thought of as a woman's remedy, although it is prescribed for men when the totality fits the case. This patient is mild, gentle and yielding; weeps easily. She is affectionate and loves sympathy and fuss. The 'typical' *Pulsatilla* has fair hair, blue eyes and rather flabby muscles. 'Changeable' is one of the great keynotes. She can be smiling one minute and crying the next. Her pains constantly change from one joint to another, from one limb to another; no two stools are alike. She cannot bear heat and to be shut in a room without air makes her feel really ill. She is much better for, and desires, fresh air. This patient cannot eat rich or fat foods, they make her ill.

Nux vomica (Poison Nut) is called the man's remedy and is one of the most irritable! He is careful and zealous, inclined to get excited or angry, can be spiteful and malicious. This patient nearly always has a sedentary occupation with its attendant difficulties, about which he gets anxious and irritable. He eats and drinks too much and wakens tired and weak and generally worse. He is a cold patient, and if he catches cold he cannot get warm no matter how near he is to the fire nor how many coats and sweaters he puts on! In classical terms, 'Great heat, whole body burning hot, especially face red and hot, yet the patient cannot move or uncover in the least without feeling chilly.' He loathes wind but feels better in wet weather.

Arsenicum album (Arsenic Trioxide). The great characteristics are restlessness, burning, prostration and midnight aggravation. No patient is more restless than one needing this remedy. He moves from chair to chair, from room to room, and if ill in bed he asks to be moved to another. He has a great mental restlessness that drives him out of bed at night. There is intense burning, particularly in acute conditions, but the burning is *ameliorated by heat*. Thirst intense, drinks often but little at one time. A very fastidious patient, cannot bear a crooked picture on the wall ...

I have given a little insight into how we get to know our remedies and what they will do for sick people. Their study becomes particularly interesting and exciting as the remedies begin to 'live' for us – the experienced homoeopath can even spot a Mr *Sulphur* arm in arm with Mrs *Calc. carb.* walking down the street!

CHAPTER 11

Homoeopathy in First Aid and Acute Conditions

Acute conditions and injuries can be treated in the home with excellent results. A full case history is necessary in chronic work, but a much simpler form is adequate when dealing with acute conditions and it is advisable to record the details as follows:

1. LOCATION – eg., if a headache, exactly where in the head is the discomfort.
2. SENSATION – this must be described accurately in the patient's own words.
3. MODALITY – worse from heat, cold, pressure, lying, sitting, walking, etc.
4. CAUSE – if known.

It should be remembered that only a very few remedies are given under each ailment and a *materia medica* is necessary when the symptoms cannot be matched accurately to any of the remedies given in these pages.

The treatment of injuries in first-aid work is simpler because fewer remedies are involved and they are, in the main, specific and can be readily memorized.

DOSE

I have indicated the required dose for the beginning of treatment in all cases, but care must be taken to study the severity of the trouble and doses adjusted accordingly. The golden rule is to stop medication as soon as improvement sets in and repeat only if the same symptoms return. If after a time there is no improvement in the patient then another remedy must be sought; this necessity will show up more quickly in a very acute case such as diarrhoea or vomiting when improvement should be observed after three or four doses, whilst twenty-four to thirty-six hours may be necessary in conditions such as indigestion or throat trouble, and longer still in constipation and rheumatism.

If after a time fresh symptoms appear, then a different remedy must be found to match the new symptoms.

The pills should be taken into the mouth and placed under the tongue where they will dissolve very quickly. The remedy will thus be absorbed into the blood-stream.

TREATMENTS

ABSCESS

Belladonna 6 two pills hourly for a threatening abscess with redness, pain and throbbing.
Apis 6 two pills hourly when there is much swelling with stinging pain; there may be, in addition, redness, burning and throbbing.
Hepar sulph. 6 two pills three-hourly when matter has formed.
Silica 6 three-hourly when suppuration has taken place but the poison is slow to come away.
Hot fomentations should be applied every two or three hours of a teaspoonful of Calendula ø to half a pint of hot water. When the abscess has started to drain, the fomentations should be reduced to two or three times daily
(ø is the sign for a homoeopathic tincture.)

ACCIDENTS – *see* INJURIES AND WOUNDS

ACNE

Carbo veg. 6 every six hours for simple and recent acne in young people.
Belladonna 6 every six hours with florid complexion.
Pulsatilla 3 every four hours if pale.
Chronic acne should be treated by a qualified homoeopath.

ANXIETY, GRIEF, WORRY, effects of
Ignatia 30 three times daily for three to five days according to the severity.
Mag. Carb. 200 three times daily for two to three days.

BACKACHE
Arnica 6 every three hours when aching is from over-exertion; for example, spring-cleaning or playing tennis for the first time.
Aesculus hip. 6 every six hours if backache with piles.
Kali carb. 6 every six hours in pregnant women with a sense of weakness in the back.
Rhus. tox. 6 or 12 every three hours for muscular stiffness from over-exertion or exposure to cold and wet.

BILIOUS OR STOMACH UPSETS
Iris versicolor 6 every two hours for nausea and vomiting of sour fluid that excoriates the throat. Sour vomit with headache. Vomiting of food an hour after eating.
Bryonia 6 or 12 every two hours when stomach is distended, with vomiting after eating. Patient must lie still, worse movement, nausea on sitting up.
Nux vomica 6 or 12 every two hours for bad effects of coffee, alcoholic drinks, debauchery. Must loosen clothing. Vomiting of food. Stomach sensitive to pressure. Patient is irritable and often cold.
Natrum sulph. 6 or 12 every two hours for constant rising of sour water. Nausea and vomiting with colic. Vomit sour followed by bitter liquids. Squeamishness in stomach before meals.
Pulsatilla 6 or 12 every four hours after fat or rich food.

BLADDER IRRITABLE
Apis 6 every two hours for frequent desire to pass water or increased in quantity and slightly burning.
Cantharis 6 every two hours for constant desire to urinate but only a few drops voided.

Causticum 6 every six hours for involuntary passage of urine on coughing or sneezing.
Other bladder symptoms should be referred to a qualified homoeopath.

BOILS

Gunpowder 3X three tablets every three hours when there are no special indications.
Belladonna 6 every two hours when a boil is just beginning to form.
Silica 6 every six hours should be given when more advanced and pus is forming.
Arnica 6 every eight hours will act as a preventive when there is a tendency to boils.

BRAIN-FAG

Phos. acid 6 or 12 three times daily. Nervous prostration. Tired mentally and physically.
Kali Phos. 12 three times daily. Weak and tired. Want of nerve power. Brain-fag with hysteria; extreme lassitude and depression. Works especially well on young people.
Anacardium 12 three times daily. Loss of memory; funk before an examination.
Calc. phos. 6 or 12 three times daily. Brain weakness after much worry or following an illness.
Silica 6 or 12 three times daily. Chronic headaches, nervousness, loss of memory from overwork; worse from cold and better warmth.

BRONCHITIS

Aconite 6 every six hours at the onset when there are chills, fever, oppression, dry, tickling cough.
Bryonia 6 every six hours when fever is established, the cough is dry, hacking or with only a little mucus; hoarseness; pains between shoulders, sharp pains on chest; constipation.
Belladonna 6 or 12 every two hours for short, dry cough

with tickling in the larynx; dry spasmodic cough with vomiting; stitches in chest; headache; redness and heat of face.

Mercurius sol. 3 every three hours for spasmodic cough; worse evening and night; tickling in chest, feels dry. Copious sweating without relief – the more he sweats the worse he feels.

Ipecacuanha 6 hourly for oppression of chest; great depression; cough and hoarseness; much expectoration, clear or white. This remedy is commonly indicated in bronchitis of children.

A qualified homoeopath should be consulted if the patient does not respond very quickly.

BRUISES

Arnica 12 hourly when bruising of soft parts.

Ruta 12 every two hours when bruising of bones.

Bellis Perennis 6 every two hours when bruising of female breast.

Conium 12 every two hours to follow *Bellis* if necessary.

Hypericum 6 every two hours when bruising of parts rich in nerves (fingers, toes, coccyx).

BURNS

Urtica urens 30 and ø should be in every kitchen. When cooking it is so easy to burn one's hand or arm on the stove, or with steam from a saucepan or kettle. Very often applying the tincture at once is all that is necessary, but if pain soon returns then a dose of the 30th potency will remove it. More tincture may be applied and the internal dose may be repeated as and when required. Of course, any burns can be treated in this way, but if very serious then a doctor should be called in.

CARBUNCLE

Anthracinum 30 every two to four hours will often abort the case.

Belladonna 6 every two hours if there is heat, redness, throbbing and swelling.
Apis 6 every two hours with oedema and swelling of tissue around.
Tarentula cubensis 30 two-hourly with burning and stinging pains.
Silica 6 every eight hours after the carbuncle has begun to discharge.
Calendula ointment may be used as a dressing.

CATARRH

Bryonia 6 or 12, a dose every three hours for catarrh extending to front sinuses or into the chest. Offensive smell from mouth with hawking of offensive, tough mucus, sometimes in round, cheesy lumps the size of a pea.
Calcarea carb. 6 or 12, a dose every four hours when nose is obstructed by yellow, fetid pus. Nostrils sore and ulcerated. At night nose dry and obstructed; by day it is moist and free. Catarrhal symptoms accompanied by great hunger.
Hepar sulph. 6 or 12 every three hours – thick, yellow, offensive catarrh with inflamed swelling of nose which is painful; also pressure on larynx; hoarseness.
Kali bichromicum 6 or 12 every three hours. Catarrh with thick yellow or greenish ropy, stringy mucus (can be pulled out in long strings) or tough and jellylike, offensive. Distress and fullness from inflammation in frontal sinuses.
Mercurius sol. 6 or 12 every three hours. Catarrhal inflammation of frontal sinuses, nasal bones swollen. Greenish fetid mucus. This remedy should be taken by those with a general tendency to catarrh three times daily for two or three weeks, repeating at intervals.
Natrum muriaticum 6 or 12 every three hours. Mucus thick and like the white of an egg. There is much sneezing. Patients needing this remedy are often chilly and constipated and love salt.
Pulsatilla 6 or 12 every four hours. Green, fetid nasal dis-

charge with diminished taste. In chronic catarrh thick, yellow, bland mucus. Better in the open air. Nose stuffs up at night and indoors but fluent in open air. Loss of smell with catarrh. Patients needing this remedy are often tearful and they feel better in themselves when walking in the air.

CHICKEN POX

Aconite 6 every two hours in the early stages with restlessness, anxiety and high fever.

Antimonium tart. 6 or 12 every two hours when vesicles form.

Rhus. tox. 6 every two hours if there is intense itching. Very often this is the only remedy required and when administered the symptoms soon disappear. When chicken pox breaks out in the home or at school, those not infected should take one dose of *rhus. tox.* 6 nightly for six nights.

CHILBLAINS

Pulsatilla 6 every six hours when there is a tendency to chilblains; patients with irritable skins; more painful when hot; in girls with painful or scanty menses.

Agaricus 6 three-hourly when chilblains are more painful when cold.

Rhus. tox. 6 every six hours if dusky red and much burning.

Petroleum 6 every three hours if broken and *Calendula* ointment applied.

Tamus ø applied locally with a brush night and morning is helpful.

Tamus ointment rubbed in night and morning at very first sign of a chilblain will often abort the trouble.

CIRCULATION FEEBLE

Frequent and regular walking in fresh air is extremely important. Sponging with tepid water in which sea-salt has been dissolved followed by rapid friction is very helpful.

Rhus. tox. 6 every four hours when there is blueness of skin.

Natrum mur. 6 every eight hours – coldness of hands and feet; unhealthy complexion.
Calc. carb. 6 or 12 every eight hours – cold hands and feet, legs feel as if damp stockings on legs.
Silica 12 every eight hours. Sensitive to slightest draught of air.

COLDS

Aconite 6 or 12. A dose hourly for three doses should be given at the sudden onset from exposure to cold or to cold dry winds. Fluent coryza of clear hot water and frequent sneezing. There may be headache, fever, thirst and sleeplessness. Doses should be given at longer intervals when symptoms improve.
Allium Cepa 6 or 12. This remedy is needed when there is streaming of the eyes and nose with headache; the profuse discharge from the nose is acrid, corroding lips and nose; watering of the eyes, also profuse, is bland. Patient is hot and thirsty; worse indoors in warm room and in the evening. Better in the open air.
Arsenicum alb. 6 or 12 every two hours. This remedy clears up a cold with thin watery discharge from nose which excoriates the upper lip, but the nose feels stuffed-up all the time. Sneezing which does not relieve irritation in the nose. Head colds and sneezing from changes in the weather which often go down on the chest. Patient is chilly, likes to be near the fire, cannot get warm in spite of many clothes. He is restless, anxious and fastidious.
Bryonia 6 or 12 every two hours. Cold begins with a running nose, sneezing and watering, aching eyes and headache on first day; then it begins to travel downwards to throat and larynx with hoarseness; bronchitis may develop.
Camphor ø at the very onset when a person is thoroughly chilled and cannot get warm; two drops on a lump of sugar and repeated until warm will often abort a cold.
Dulcamara 6 or 12 every two hours is excellent for colds

from cold, wet weather and snow; from getting wet or chilled when heated. Profuse discharge of water from nose and eyes, worse in open air, more fluent indoors in the warm, less fluent in cold air, or in a cold room. Sneezing worse in the cold. Eyes become red and sore.

Gelsemium 6 or 12 every two hours. Colds needing this remedy commence several days after exposure. Discharge makes nostrils sore and feel as if red-hot water is running down the nose. There are chills running up and down the back and the patient feels a great weight and tiredness of the whole body.

Nux Vomica 6 or 12 every two hours, for colds which come on in dry, cold weather. Nose is stuffed up at night and in the open air; fluent coryza in warm room and by day. Sneezing. Patient is cold, cannot get enough clothes on and wants to hug the fire. Shivering from slightest movement or contact with the open air. This patient is usually very irritable.

COLIC

Chamomilla 6 every twenty minutes for pressive pain in stomach and under short ribs. Severe painful pressure in epigastrium making patient toss about in despair.

Colchicum 6 or 12 for colic; worse eating and after flatulent food with great distention of stomach. Better bending double.

Colocynth 6 or 12 every twenty minutes for violent cutting and tearing pains concentrating in the pit of the stomach, better from hard pressure and bending double.

Dioscorea 6 or 12 every twenty minutes for frequent sharp pains and burning, better belching. Sharp cramping pain in pit of stomach, then belching of quantities of tasteless wind, better straightening up. Doses should be given at longer intervals as soon as there is an improvement in symptoms.

CONSTIPATION

Bryonia 6 three times daily when there is no desire; urging several times before results. Chronic constipation with headache. Stools hard, dark and dry as if burnt; large stools. Abdomen distended; rumbling yet obstinate constipation. The *bryonia* patient is worse for movement and irritable. He is thirsty.

China 6 every four hours when there is accumulation of faeces in rectum.

Hydrastis 6 every six hours when there is no desire for stool; constipation alternating with looseness of bowels; with headache; after abuse of purgatives; with foul tongue; with piles.

Magnesia mur. 6 or 12 three times daily for constipation at the seaside. One of the key-notes of this remedy is worse for taking salt, and the salt in the air by the sea causes constipation. Stools dry, they crumble at anus.

Natrum mur. 6 three times daily. There is obstinate retention of stools, irregular, hard and dry, often on alternate days. Does not know whether flatus or stool escapes. Constipation during periods. The *natrum mur.* patient is irritable, weepy, hates fuss and craves salt.

Nux vomica 6 three times daily. There is urging for stool but it does not come. Sometimes a small stool is passed followed by a sensation that more is left behind; as if evacuation is incomplete. This remedy is often indicated for sedentary workers who are studious, extremely sensitive and very irritable.

Sepia 6 every four hours for ineffectual urging, stool not hard but much straining and sometimes sweating. Constipation of pregnancy. Feeling of a ball in the rectum which is not relieved by stool. Prolapse. The *sepia* patient is dull and indifferent with a tendency to prolapse, a feeling of heaviness and sagging.

Sulphur 6 every eight hours for stool only every two or three days which is hard, large and difficult. There is sometimes a sensation as if something is left behind in the rectum (like nux. vom.) and there may be piles that bleed. The *sulphur* patient is warm, puts feet out of bed and throws off the clothes. He is hungry mid-morning.

Two tablespoonsful of bran night and morning has cured many cases of constipation. The amount should be adjusted for individual needs.

COUGHS

Aconite 6 or 12 every three hours for constant short, dry cough with no expectoration; comes on suddenly after exposure to cold, dry winds. Wakens patient from sleep, dry, croupy and suffocating. Patient is anxious, fearful and restless. Worse at night.

Bryonia 6 or 12 every three hours for a hard, dry cough with soreness in chest. Worse at night, after eating and drinking, and when entering a warm room. Cough compels patient to spring out of bed. Goes down to chest. Irritable patient.

Calc. carb. 6 every two hours. Cough from tickling as if from feather in throat; constant tickle causing a hacking cough; cough during and after eating.

Causticum 6 or 12 for hard cough which hurts whole chest. Inability to expectorate, patient feels if he could cough a little deeper he could bring up the mucus. Urine often escapes when coughing. Voice almost gone.

Pulsatilla 6 or 12 every three hours. Cough caused by inspiration. Worse warm room or coming into a warm room. Cough in the evening, worse lying down, prevents sleep. Paroxysmal cough from tickling in larynx. Dry cough, wants doors and windows open. Mucus thick, bland, yellowish-green.

Rumex 6 or 12 every three hours for cough from breathing cool air; from changing to cold from warmth. Much tough mucus in larynx and constant desire to hawk without relief. Hoarseness. Dry spasmodic cough.

Spongia 6 or 12 every three hours. Croupy cough, sounds like a saw being driven through a board, with loss of voice. Chest dry. Wakens feeling suffocated with loud, violent cough, anxiety and difficult breathing. Cough worse talking, reading, singing, swallowing and lying with head low.

CRAMP

Arnica 6 every two hours if cramp is in the calves from fatigue.
Cuprum 6 for contractions of muscles and tendons – a dose as is necessary and three times daily for a week following an attack.
Ledum 12 is excellent and often the only remedy necessary. Should be taken every ten minutes for three doses and three times daily for a week following an attack.
Nux vomica 6 every eight hours if cramp is from no special cause, coming on at night. May be repeated in the night if necessary.

DANDRUFF *see* HAIR

DEBILITY

If this is a symptom of present disease then it is this disease that must be cleared up.
Calc. phos. 6 every eight hours – debility and exhaustion from overwork or worry.
Psorinum 30 three times daily for three days after acute diseases; prostration, chilliness and desire to lie down.
Ferrum phos. 6 every eight hours – debility with flushes of head and face; brain feels tired.
Mag. carb. 200 three times daily for three days in overwrought, nervously run-down women.
Nux vomica 6 three times daily – irritability, weakness, loss of appetite, constipation.
Calc. carb. 6 every eight hours for debility in fat, pale children.
Silica 6 every eight hours for debility in thin, rickety children.
China 3 or 6 every six hours for debility from loss of blood or other animal fluids; from overwork or anxiety.

A VISIT TO THE DENTIST

Gelsemium 30, a dose an hour before and a second dose just before going to the dentist calms the agitated person who gets worked up and sometimes develops diarrhoea.
Arnica 30 should be taken as soon after leaving the surgery as possible after extractions or fillings. Another dose or two may follow according to the severity of the treatment.

DIARRHOEA

Camphor ø, two drops on sugar, will often clear up acute diarrhoea if repeated every fifteen minutes.
Phos. acid 6 hourly when diarrhoea is painless, greyish-white, watery, involuntary; evacuations not followed by feeling of weakness.
Aloe 6 every two hours when there is sense of insecurity in rectum, uncertain whether gas or stool will come.
Colocynth 6 every two hours when there are brown, watery stools after eating or drinking with much colic.
Arsenicum alb. 6 or 12, hourly for three doses and less often as improvement begins for relentless purging often with vomiting; diarrhoea after eating ices or taking cold drinks when hot. Also after tainted meat, food or fruit.
Bryonia 6 or 12, every hour for three doses and less often as symptoms improve for diarrhoea in hot weather; vomits food; colic with thirst for long drinks; lumpy diarrhoea. Dry, parched lips.
China 6 or 12, hourly for three doses and less often when symptoms improve for watery diarrhoea with much flatus; passes undigested food. Very debilitating.
Dulcamara 6 or 12, hourly for three doses and less often when symptoms improve for sudden attacks of diarrhoea in cold, wet weather, every change of weather to cool. Colic as if diarrhoea would occur.
Podophyllum 6 or 12, hourly for three doses and less often as symptoms improve for profuse stools, offensive, gushing, painless. Desire for water but not for food.

DYSPEPSIA – *see* INDIGESTION

EARACHE

Aconite 6 every hour for earache from cold.
Pulsatilla 6 every hour follows *Aconite* well if the symptom is not completely cleared up.
Chamomilla 6, hourly when pain seems intolerable; is worse for warmth and at night.
Verbascum oil, one or two drops in the ear will generally relieve the pain very quickly.

FEET ACHING

Arnica 30, hourly for two or three doses when aching from over-walking.
Arnica ø, a teaspoonful in a bowl of water is very comforting when feet are bathed. This can be refreshing in hot weather.

GUM-BOILS

Merc. sol. 6 every two hours.

HAIR TROUBLES

Arsenicum alb. 6 every six hours when there is dry scurf.
Bryonia 6 every eight hours for very greasy hair.
Fluoric Acid 4 every four hours for dry, scurfy, irritable scalp; falling of hair.
Kali carb. 6 every six hours when hair is very dry or when dry and falling out.
Phosphoric acid 6 every six hours for hair falling out from depressing emotions.
Sepia 6 every six hours for moist scurf.
Sulphur 30 every six hours for thick scurf.

HAEMORRHOIDS (Piles)

Aesculus hip. 6 every four hours where there is much uneasiness, pain in back, constipation, general absence of bleeding, but pain like sticks in rectum. Worse walking.

Causticum 6 or 12 every eight hours for hard piles, very painful when touched, walking, standing or sitting; better after a stool. Itching, stitching, stinging, burning and moist.

Hamamelis 3 every four hours for bleeding piles with loose stools. The rectum should be bathed with 30 drops of hamamelis ø in half a pint of water night and morning.

Nitric Acid 6 or 12 every four hours for piles which protrude and often bleed; burning and itching of anus; cutting pain after stool, constipation.

Nux vomica 3 every eight hours for blind piles in persons of sedentary life, of costive habits.

Sulphur 6, eight-hourly for bleeding piles, costiveness, feeling of faintness, sinking sensation mid-morning; worse at night on getting warm in bed and from washing.

HAY FEVER

Chrome Alum. 3x every four hours covers a large majority of cases, and is equally protective if taken before the season begins.

Allium cepa. 12, hourly when there is copious and acrid discharge; eyes watery; burning in eyelids; catarrhal; symptoms worse indoors, better in open air.

Sabadilla 6 every four hours for violent sneezing, redness and swelling of eyelids, with headache.

Mixed Pollens 30 three times daily for three or four days will clear up the condition if it is ascertained that the patient is allergic to pollens.

Mixed Grasses 30 three times daily for three or four days will clear up the condition if it is ascertained that the patient is allergic to grasses.

HEADACHES

Two pills at hourly intervals may be given for the first three or four doses and then less often as improvement sets in.

Arsenicum alb. 6 every two hours – burning sensation on

top of head; periodical headache accompanied by or arising from debility.

Bryonia 6 or 12 for bursting or splitting headaches worse from any motion. Cannot sit up in bed. Worse any movement. Better lying still.

Gelsemium 6 or 12 for congestive headaches, pulsating. Neuralgic headache in temples and over the eyes, with nausea. Relieved by copious urination. Lies with head high, feels exhausted.

Glonoine 6 or 12 for waves of terrible bursting, pulsating pain, worse bending head backwards. A good remedy for sunstroke. Worse for having hair cut. Worse heat about head. Throbbing head; head hot, face flushed.

Natrum muriaticum 6 or 12 for chronic headaches like little hammers in the head on slightest motion. Often begins at 10 or 11 am and lasts until 3 pm or evening. Better for sleep. If very acute give *Bryonia* (it's acute) first and *Natrum muriaticum* when the violent pain is over.

Nux vomica 6 or 12 for headaches of sedentary persons; better when head is wrapped up. Feels as if a nail has been driven through brain. Stabbing pain with nausea and vomiting. Headache on waking; after eating.

Pulsatilla 6 or 12 for throbbing, congestive headaches, head hot, better cold applications. Better slowly walking in fresh air. Periodic sick headaches. Headaches from over-eating. Headaches connected with menses or from suppressed menstruation.

See also MIGRAINE HEADACHES

HEARTBURN – *see* INDIGESTION

INDIGESTION

Bryonia 6 or 12 every two hours for feeling of a stone in the stomach, sharp pain through to back of chest; pain between shoulders; bilious vomiting; pain across forehead; white tongue; constipation.

Calcarea carb. 6 every six hours when there is ravenous hunger, white-coated tongue; heartburn; waterbrash; milk disagrees; tight clothes unbearable; abdomen distended and hard; offensive white stools.

Carbo veg. 6. Great distension of the abdomen with gas; belching with sour, disordered stomach, constant eructations, flatulence, heartburn, waterbrash. Great accumulation of flatus in stomach, all food turns to wind. Relief from belching, constant belching.

Kali bich. 6 every three hours for vomiting from chronic catarrh of stomach; tongue with yellow coating; weight rather than pain after food.

Lycopodium 6. Pressure and discomfort in stomach after eating a *little* food. Must loosen clothing. Acidity, waterbrash, heartburn, fullness, flatulence, distension and bloating of stomach.

Typically this patient craves sweets and hot drinks, is worse from 4 to 8 pm. Anticipates events such as speaking in public but is all right as soon as he begins.

Natrum carb. 6. Greedy person who love sweets and nibbling. Much flatulence, always belching. Stomach sour. All-gone feeling and pain in stomach which drives him to eat.

Nux vomica 6. After a meal flatulent distension. Nausea after eating, eructations of bitter and sour food. Flatulence rises and presses under short ribs. Putrid or bitter taste in mouth but food and drink taste all right. Irritable patient.

Pulsatilla 6. From eating fat food; nausea with little vomiting; heartburn; feeling of distension, clothes have to be loosened. Patient is often weepy and is better in fresh air.

Two pills three times daily after meals in all cases.

INFLUENZA

Aconite 6 or 12. Sudden onset with fever; great restlessness from anxiety, sometimes with rapid heart beats and dry, painful cough. This medicine is needed when these symptoms come on after being out in very cold weather or cold winds.

Arsenicum alb. 6 or 12 when patient has a bad headache, teasing cough which is worse at night, is restless with anguish and very fearful. Very often there is a high temperature.

Baptisia 6 or 12. Gastric flu, sudden attacks of diarrhoea and vomiting with great prostration. Face has a dark, patchy flush; patient is dull and confused and falls asleep while answering. Aching in all limbs; headache; restlessness.

Belladonna 6 or 12 every two hours when there is headache, sore throat, teasing, tickling cough; worse lying down; delirium; neuralgia especially on right side of face and head; inflammation of ears.

Bryonia 6 or 12. The outstanding symptom of patients needing this remedy is that they do not want to move; they are worse from movement and want to be left alone and resent being disturbed. Thirst for long drinks of cold fluid at long intervals. Mouth and lips parched; dry hacking cough hurts the chest and head. Patient is irritable.

Gelsemium 6 or 12. The onset of flu calling for this remedy is gradual – perhaps two or three days. Patient looks drowsy with heavy eyelids, heavy head and heavy limbs. He is a tired patient. Chills run up and down back and during the fever there is no thirst. There is pain on moving the eyes and bursting headache from neck over head to eyes and forehead which is better by copious urination.

Eupatorium perf. 6 or 12. Intense aching in the bones of limbs and back, patient dare not move for pain. There is bursting headache, shivering, chills, vomiting of bile after drinking; great thirst, nausea, sneezing, soreness of eyeballs, watering eyes, hacking cough and hoarseness.

Remedies for influenza may be taken at hourly intervals for the first three or four doses and then at longer intervals as improvement sets in.

INJURIES

Arnica 30, hourly for up to three doses and then frequently according to the severity for bruising from falls, blows, accidents, and for the shock which follows.

Bumps on the heads of children should be bathed with liberal amounts of cold water, or water to which has been added a few drops of *Arnica* ø (mother tincture), and *Arnica* 30 given internally. Note: *Arnica* tincture must never be applied to open wounds where the skin is broken.

'Bruised and sore' describes the damage which *Arnica* will remove.

Rhus. tox. 12 or 30 for sprains and strains of muscles, tendons and ligaments, particularly when the injured part is relieved by an application of heat in any form. This follows *Arnica* well, and the same instructions regarding dosage apply.

Ruta 6 or 12 is indicated for injuries of the periosteum (membrane covering the bone), for pain as if bruised in the bones, for bruised bones and for wounds where bones are injured. Sometimes relief is not obtained from *Arnica*, and then the involvement of the bones reveals itself. This remedy should be given three times daily for at least a week, according to the severity of the trouble.

Symphytum 30 once daily for two weeks is a remedy to facilitate the union of fractured bones by favouring formation of callus; the pain at the seat of the injury is pricking and stitching. This remedy will also relieve the irritability of stumps after amputation, and it will clear up periosteal pains after the wounds have healed.

Calendula has great healing properties and should be used for all lacerated wounds, dental lacerations, and any torn or jagged wound. It quickly heals lacerated gums after teeth extractions.

In any laceration the wound should be washed in a solution of one part *Calendula* to ten of water. It is beneficial also to take *Calendula* in the 30th potency internally every three hours for one or two days according to the severity, to promote healing.

Hamamelis 30, half-hourly for up to three doses and then less often when there are sore, painful, incised, lacerated, contused wounds with much bleeding. This remedy checks the bleeding, removes the pain and promotes rapid healing. It is a valuable haemorrhage remedy.

Hypericum 12 or 30. This remedy will soothe the intense pain caused by injury to sentient nerves; from stepping on nails, tacks, pins, from splinters, or from the bite of an animal. When the pain travels upwards from the seat of the injury and threatens tetanus (lock-jaw); where the finger ends, after being shut in a door, or the toes, have been bruised and lacerated, or a nail torn off, or a splinter run under the nail; if the pain travels upwards from the seat of the injury along the nerve towards the body, *Hypericum* should be administered at once and repeated at half-hourly intervals until the pain lessens and the wound becomes more comfortable. *Tetanus from wounds will not develop if* Hypericum *is given.* Injuries to the spine such as a fall on the coccyx, or concussion of the spine when the whole spine is very sensitive to touch, will respond well to *Hypericum.* The coccyx has many nerve endings, and even if the injury was sustained long before homoeopathic treatment is administered, *Hypericum* will still give relief.

Ledum 12 or 30 should be administered for 'puncture' wounds – wounds from nails, pointed instruments; from stepping on tacks, from running the garden fork through the foot, from puncturing with needles and running splinters into the flesh or under the nails. These are very much like the wounds listed under *Hypericum*, but when the injured part *feels cold, is puffed, pale and mottled,* give *Ledum.*

Ledum 200 is a routine remedy for black eye. This will remove pain and discoloration quickly. One dose should be given and a second one only if necessary.

INSOMNIA

Arnica 30, a dose at bedtime when physically overtired; body aches, cannot get comfortable, the bed feels hard.
Aconite 6 or 12, three doses at half-hourly intervals at bedtime when there is anxiety, restlessness and patient is fearful. Sleeplessness of aged people; anxious dreams.
Arsenicum alb. 6 or 12, three doses at hourly intervals at bedtime, for sleeplessness with anxiety and restlessness, tossing around the bed, cannot keep legs still.
Coffea 6 or 12, three doses at half-hourly intervals at bedtime for sleeplessness from agitation, thoughts crowding into the mind, usually patient is worried.
There is every chance that one dose of the indicated remedy will prove successful so the mind should not be conditioned to the maximum number of doses. However, if sleep proves difficult to capture, the indicated remedy should be taken three times daily for a week to ten days, the last dose being taken at bedtime.

LUMBAGO

Aconite 6 or 12 every two hours during the first day, then less often as symptoms improve. Pain sharp as if beaten or sprained, from cold, dry winds; from draughts. Lumbar region very sensitive.
Aesculus hip. 3 every two hours for severe, dull, aching pain making walking, stooping and rising from sitting almost impossible, often accompanied by constipation and piles.
Arnica 6 or 12 every two hours if from an injury. Back feels as if beaten.
Antimonium tart. 6 or 12 three times daily. Backache as from fatigue especially after eating and while sitting. Violent pain in sacro-lumbar region, the slightest effort to move causes retching and cold clammy sweat. Sensation of weight hanging on coccyx and dragging downwards.
Bryonia 6 or 12 every three hours. Pain worse from every

movement, muscles painful to touch; bruised feeling in lower back when lying on it; worse from dry cold.

Rhus. tox. 6 or 12 every three hours for pains in small of back, better lying on something hard. Stiffness painful on motion; pain bruised or burning, better during motion. Worse from damp, cold.

This remedy has the characteristic of stiffness and pains being worse on first movement, but better after limbering up.

MEASLES

Aconite 6 every two hours when there is catarrh and high fever before the rash appears; subsequently itching, burning skin, rash rough, restless, anxious, tossing about, frightened.

Pulsatilla 12 every three hours when there is little fever, catarrhal symptoms, profuse lachrymation, dry mouth but seldom thirsty.

Euphrasia 6 or 12 every two hours when there is running from nose, streaming, burning tears, throbbing headache, dry cough and rash.

When measles break out in the home or school those not infected should take a dose of *Pulsatilla* 12 nightly for six nights.

MENSTRUATION DIFFICULTIES

Aconite 6 or 12 three times daily for two or three weeks when period is late, diminished but too protracted. Plethoric females who live a sedentary life. Periods suppressed by fright with vexation.

Calcarea carb. 6 or 12, three times daily for two to three weeks when period is too early, lasts too long and is too profuse, induced by mental excitement or working too hard. Suppressed menses after working in water.

Natrum muriaticum 6 or 12, three times daily for two to three weeks. Menses too late and scanty, or too early and profuse. Before menses anxious, sad, qualmish; sweetish eructations in the morning; headache, eyes heavy, palpitation. During menses headache, sadness, colic. After menses headache.

Pulsatilla 6 or 12, three times daily for two or three weeks when menses are delayed and scanty, irregular, patient pale, languid and chilly. When periods do not appear at puberty and there is no local or constitutional disease to account for it.

Sabina 6, three times daily for two or three weeks. Menses too profuse, too early; flow in paroxysms; with colic and labour pains.

Sepia 6 or 12, three times daily for two or three weeks. Menses too early and too profuse; too late and too scanty; suppressed.

MIGRAINE HEADACHES

Capsicum 6 every hour for bursting headache, full, constant, pressing pain above the root of the nose, together with stitches through and over the eye; stitching headache; throbbing in one or other temple; drawing, tearing headache.

Ignatia 12 every two hours when there is pressive aching in spots; pressure at centre of forehead and root of nose; headache from worry, anxiety or grief; pressing, sick headache with disturbance of vision passing off with copious discharge of clear urine.

Iris vers. 12 or 30, hourly for three doses then less often. Sick headache, worse rest; begins with a blur before the eyes; frontal headache with nausea.

Kali bich. 6 every two hours – headache over one eye, especially the right; before headache comes on there is blurred vision, the sight improving when the pain begins.

Kali carb. 6 half-hourly. Drawing, tearing, pressing pains; intolerance of light; disturbance of vision.

Onosmodium 12 two-hourly. Head feels dull, heavy, pain pressing upward in occiput. Occiputal-frontal pain in morning on waking, chiefly left side. Dizziness, vision blurred.

Sanguinaria 6, every two hours for one-sided sick headache, pain coming from back of head and settling in right eye; worse lying down and sleeping; accompanied by bilious vomiting. Electric shooting in head; shivering; (menses profuse).

MUMPS

Jaborandi 6 or 12 every two hours. Should be given at the beginning of all cases of mumps as it so often clears up the symptoms and removes the pain before any complications set in.
Aconite 6 or 12 every two hours when there is fever, thirst and anxiety plus pain.
Carbo veg. 6 or 12 every three hours if the patient catches cold during mumps and the mammary glands are affected in girls or the testicles in boys.
Mercurius cor. 6 every two hours following *Aconite* when fever has subsided.
Pulsatilla 6 or 12 every three hours if the testicles become affected and are swollen.
When mumps break out in the home or at school, all those not infected should take *Jaborandi* 6 at bedtime for six nights.

NAILS

Silica 6 every six hours – nails brittle and powdery when cut, rough and yellow.
Thuja 6 every eight hours – crippled, discoloured and crumbling nails.
Alumina 6 every eight hours – brittle nails, thick spots on them. Brittle skin on finger-tips.
Graphites 6 every six hours when nails are thick or corrugated.

NERVOUS CONDITIONS – *see* SHOCK AND NERVOUS CONDITIONS

NOSE BLEEDING

Millefolium 30 every half an hour – in general.
Arnica 30 every fifteen minutes when from a blow.
Bryonia 3 every fifteen minutes – bright red blood on getting up in the morning. Can be taken three times daily for a few days as a preventive.
Ferrum phos. 6 every eight hours for recurrent bleeding without appreciable cause.
Carbo veg. 6 every eight hours for recurrent bleeding in old people.

OPERATIONS

Gelsenium 30. If worked-up beforehand, a dose at bedtime the previous night and another dose on waking on morning of operation. A third dose is permitted if necessary and if there is time.
Arnica 30 should be taken as soon after the operation as possible, followed by three doses daily for three days.

PILES – *see* HAEMORRHOIDS

RHEUMATISM

Arnica 12, three times daily for two to three weeks for articular or muscular rheumatism, from exposure to dampness and cold; strained muscles due to over-exertion. Limbs ache as if beaten; affected parts feel sore and bruised.
Bryonia 6 or 12 every four hours for heaviness of the limbs; they feel like lead (especially the lower), with redness and swelling of joints. Weakness of limbs compels patient to sit down. Worse on movement.
Caulophyllum 6 every two hours when small joints of hands and feet are affected.
Colchicum 6 or 12 three times daily for two or three weeks for rheumatism in the small joints, tearing pains in muscles and joints.

Kali bich. 6 every six hours – chronic rheumatism, tearing pains about the joints.

Rhododendron 6 every two hours – muscular and fibrous tissues affected; from exposure to dry cold; worse stormy weather.

Ruta 6 two-hourly – joints and neighbouring bones painful; cold non-inflammatory affections, especially wrists and ankles.

Rhus. tox. 6 or 12 three times daily for two or three weeks for swelling and stiffness of joints from sprains, over-lifting or over-stretching. Pains in limbs with numbness and tingling; joints weak or stiff; shining swelling of joints. Worse on beginning to move and in wet, damp weather. Better from continued motion. Tearing pains in limbs during rest.

SCIATICA

Amon. mur. 6 every two hours for pain worse sitting, somewhat relieved by walking, entirely by lying down; sensation as if hamstring muscles were too short.

Capsicum 6 every four hours for shooting, tearing from hip to knee and foot.

Gnaphalium 6 every two hours for intense pain in the nerve accompanied by cramps, or alternating with numbness.

Lycopodium 12 every four hours when pain is right-sided, worse afternoon, worse lying on affected side or by least touch.

Mag. phos. 12 every two hours – lightning-like pains, right side, better warmth.

Rhus. tox. 6 every two hours. Pain worse in bed at night or when at rest.

SEA-SICKNESS

Petroleum 6 every eight hours. In general give for two days before going on board and one- to two-hourly when the voyage begins.

Cocculus 6 every six hours when there is vertigo and empty feeling in head with nausea and vomiting. Give for a few days before voyage and hourly during.

Tabacum 30 every six hours for two or three days prior to voyage and half-hourly if sea-sickness develops with prostration and cold sweat.

Borax 30 hourly when the downward motion is most felt.

SHOCK AND NERVOUS CONDITIONS

Arnica 30. Shock from accidents or physical injuries. Please note that this remedy will not deal with shock from any other cause.

Aconite 12. Shock from fear; it steadies the nervous system. (This remedy helped many people during the air-raids of the last war.)

Ignatia 30. Shock from grief or fright, often with hysterical weeping and sometimes with fainting. It has helped many people after the death of a loved one.

Gelsemium 12. Nervous symptoms anticipating some event (like going to the dentist); examination funk; there is agitation, trembling and a feeling of limpness. In all cases a dose should be taken at once, followed by one or two more at half-hourly or hourly intervals according to severity.

SLEEPLESSNESS – *see* INSOMNIA

STIFF NECK

Aconite 6 every hour when stiffness is from a draught or chill; tearing in the nape, painful stiff neck.

Actea Racemosa 6 every hour when head and neck are retracted; rheumatic pain and stiffness in muscles of neck and back, sensitiveness of spine.

Bryonia 6 every hour for painful stiff neck worse from touch or motion.

Dulcamara 6 every hour when stiffness is from damp or cold. Pain in neck as after lying with head in uncomfortable position.

Rhododendron 6 every hour when trouble is from dry, cold; pain worse on approach of stormy weather.

STINGS OF BEES AND WASPS

Urtica urens 30 every two hours.
Apis 30 every five minutes if there are symptoms of collapse in bee or wasp stings. If ammonia is not available the sting may be covered with a slice of onion which is very efficacious.

STINGS OF INSECTS

Ledum 6 every ten minutes and Ledum ø may be painted on the part, or ammonia applied.

STOMACH UPSETS – *see* BILIOUS AND STOMACH UPSETS

STYES

Pulsatilla 6 every two hours at the onset.
Staphysagria 6 every two hours to follow *Pulsatilla* if necessary.
Hepar sulph. 6 every four hours in chronic cases and for tendency to styes.

TEETHING BABIES

Chamomilla 6 is a wonderful remedy when a baby is teething, especially when one cheek is red and he is crying; does not know what he wants; as soon as you give him a toy he throws it down and wants something else. This remedy soothes and calms and has restored sleep to many parents in the middle of the night.
Dissolve three or four pills in a quarter of a tumbler of warm water and give a teaspoonful as a dose every twenty minutes until the baby is calm or asleep.

THROAT TROUBLES

Aconite 6 or 12. Throat very red, tingling. Acute

inflammation which comes on suddenly (often in the night) after exposure to cold, raw wind.

Baryta carb. 6 or 12. Every exposure to damp or cold brings on a sore throat with inflammation of tonsils, throat and fauces. It is slow to develop. Children with large tonsils who are intellectually retarded benefit from this remedy.

Belladonna 6. Inflammation of the throat; fauces and tonsils bright red and inflamed, especially right side, sometimes extending to left. Painful to swallow. Dryness of fauces. Aversion to liquids.

Patients needing this remedy nearly always have a congested, red, hot face and skin. Heat and dryness are marked.

Dulcamara 6 or 12. Sore throat from damp, cold weather; tendency to ulceration. Catarrh. Throat fills with mucus. Tonsils inflamed.

Kali bich. 6 or 12. Tonsils swollen and inflamed; ulcers which tend to perforate. Discharges ropy, stringy and yellow which stick like glue.

Mercurius sol. 6 or 12. Sore throat with every cold, smarting, raw. Discharge from nose yellowy-green, thick mucus. Tongue thick, moist covering. Much sweating without relief. Worse at night.

Nux vomica 6 or 12. Sore throat; cold settles in nose, throat, chest and ears. Sneezing from itching in nose and throat. Sensitive to least draught. Patient is burning and hot but cannot move or uncover without feeling chilly. Often irritable.

Pulsatilla 6 or 12. Catarrh affecting throat which is bluish-red. Stinging pains, worse swallowing saliva. Worse in warm air and room. Better cold, fresh, open air. Patient is sometimes weepy.

A dose of the appropriate remedy should be given every three hours until improvement sets in and then less often.

VARICOSE VEINS

Pulsatilla 3 every eight hours as a preventive or when an

attack is feared. If there is much pain in veins this remedy should be given every two hours.
Hamamelis 3 every three hours when veins are enlarged and full.
Fluoric Acid 3 every four hours for long-standing cases.
Hamamelis lotion should be applied night and morning. (30 drops of ø in half a pint of water.)

VOICE, LOSS OF

Arnica 6 every two hours when the trouble is from over-exertion.
Baryta carb. 12 every four hours for chronic hoarseness.
Causticum 6 every two hours when voice is affected by simple catarrh.
Gelsemium 6 every two hours when loss of voice is during menstrual periods.

VOMITING

Bryonia 6 or 12 hourly. Vomiting of solid food immediately after eating. Nausea and vomiting in morning when waking; worse movement.
Ipecacuanha 6 or 12 hourly. Vomiting with *constant* nausea.
Nux vomica 6 or 12 hourly. Vomiting food and drink after overloading stomach. Usually feels cold and irritable.
Pulsatilla 6 or 12 hourly. Vomiting from a cold on the stomach or suppressed menses; after eating too much fat, pastry, etc. Pale face with chilliness.
After three hourly doses longer intervals should be allowed as symptoms improve, otherwise another remedy should be given.
The cause of vomiting must be ascertained and then treated accordingly.

WARTS

Thuja 12 or 30 every four hours for warts in crops; flat, black warts; large, seedy, pedunculated, sometimes oozing moisture and bleeding readily.

Calc. carb. 6 every four hours when there are numerous small warts which are horny, itching, stinging, inflamed, or ulcerating.

Causticum 12 every eight hours when there are many small warts; soft at base, horny on surface; on hands, arms, eyelids and face.

Nitric Acid 12 every four hours when warts are itching, sticking, and prickling; large, jagged, pedunculated, easily bleeding; cauliflower-like.

WHOOPING COUGH

Arnica 6 or 12 is a wonderful remedy for a violent tickling cough which commences when a child gets angry. Begins to cry before cough; child knows it is coming and dreads it.

Bryonia 6 or 12. Child coughs immediately after eating and drinking, then vomits; he returns to finish his meal and the same thing happens again. Dry, hard, spasmodic cough. Cough makes him spring out of bed.

Carbo veg. 6 or 12. An excellent remedy to be given at the beginning of whooping cough, especially if child is fond of salt. Cough mostly hard and dry. Every violent spell brings up a lump of phlegm or is followed by retching and gagging, with very red face.

Drosera 6. Spasmodic cough with retching and vomiting. Often the only remedy required.

Kali carb. 6 or 12. Convulsive and tickling cough at night. Cough violent and causes vomiting.

A dose of the indicated remedy should be given after every spasm of coughing.

When whooping cough breaks out in the home or at school, all those not infected should take *Drosera* 6 night and morning for one week.

CHAPTER 12

Homoeopathy and Surgery

Many people think that the homoeopath is against all surgery. This, of course, is far from the truth. Surgery today is of the highest standard and I personally have the greatest regard for surgeons. What horrifies me, however, is the number of unnecessary operations that are performed.

Let us examine some of the conditions where surgery is so often employed unnecessarily. Haemorrhoids (piles) whether external or internal, whether bleeding or not, are regarded by the allopath as a purely local disturbance. If very troublesome they are removed by surgery. Unhappily, this makes the situation worse for the *cause* of the haemorrhoids is still in the economy and inevitably more trouble awaits the patient at a later date. We believe that haemorrhoids are a local manifestation of faulty portal circulation or other constitutional trouble; and we know that if they are removed surgically nature will attempt to re-establish the condition and, if unsuccessful, then trouble of a more serious nature will manifest itself in a more vital part. We prescribe the remedy most similar to the patient's entire economy, of which the haemorrhoid is only a part. Many hundreds of such cases have been completely cured because the whole man has been harmonized and the *cause* of the trouble removed.

The following case comes from the records of the late Dr Harvey Farrington, a famous American homoeopathic physician:

Mrs M.W., aged 37, stout, plethoric, excitable, has suffered from piles off and on since childhood. Her mother died of cancer of the rectum. She came to me on 19 December with the following symptoms – pain in rectum for hours after stool, whether it be hard or soft, throbbing and prickling relieved by either cold or hot applications. Headaches in the vertex with nausea. Menses three to five days early, profuse, clotted. Burning of the soles of the feet. Craves sweets of all kinds especially cakes. Much flatulence in abdomen after eating so that at times she is obliged to loosen clothing. Occasional spells of diarrhoea which drive her out of bed at 5 am. *Sulphur* relieved her for some time, and later a course of *Carbo veg.* from the thousandth to the millionth potency so ameliorated the symptoms that she stopped coming.

On the 6 October the following year she returned, saying that the same old pain had returned with doubled severity and she feared that a rectal cancer was developing. She had been told, by another homoeopath, that she would never be well unless she had an operation.

The general aspect of the case had now changed. She was more nervous and excitable than ever, characterizing her symptoms with adjectives all in the superlative. The headaches still persisted and she stated she was hungry while they lasted. Menses every three weeks. Rectal inactivity; can with great effort void a normal soft stool, but usually without pain. In an hour or so after evacuation the most horrible throbbing begins and persists for a long period of time. At various times during the day there are sharp, sticking pains which shoot upwards into the rectum. The haemorrhoids protrude after stool and at times they bleed. Pain in the rectum when coughing.

A close study of the case led to the selection of *Ignatia* which gave immediate relief in the thousandth potency.

10 December – symptoms returning; the same potency was repeated. One dose of the CM potency was given two weeks later and for several years there has been neither pain nor soreness in the rectum.

Dr Kent cites the interesting case of a man who came to see him and asked him to remove a tumour (by surgery) which had been removed twice before and was given the name 'recurrent fibroid'. It was the size of a hen's egg, very hard, located in the left side of the neck, not connected with the parotid though growing a little below it.

Dr Kent says: 'I advised him to give me a little time to prepare him for removal. I took his symptoms and found that he was better by wrapping up even his head. He was timid in going into a new enterprise though abundantly able to perform the task. *He lacked confidence in his own ability, yet when he had begun he would do well.*'

The patient was given *Silica* in high potency on 1 April. Six weeks later he called to see Dr Kent again – the tumour was reduced to half the size. He was given *Silica* in a higher potency. Six weeks later it was almost gone. On 23 January of the following year he had a third dose of the same remedy in the same potency – the tumour disappeared.

Dr Kent's comments about this case are interesting: 'The tumour was not included in the totality of symptoms as it was not a symptom; it furnished no part of the guide to a remedy. The symptoms expressive of the whole state existed prior to the tumour and it was the language of the pre-existing state that I must read, as out of that pre-existing state grew the tumour. I must interpret the language or expressions of *cause*, not *effect*. The doctor who is guided by pathology can use the knife. To use the knife is but to acknowledge one's ignorance of a method by which he can avoid cutting.'

It is not uncommon for uterine fibroids to be cleared up by means of homoeopathic medication. Again, the fibroid is a manifestation of a total effect. In 1896, Dr James Compton Burnett wrote a little book called *Organ Diseases of Women* in which he condemned surgical interference in these cases. He says: 'Having imbibed the idea of curing enlargements and displacements of the uterus by medicines given in the ordinary way by mouth, and having succeeded well in so doing, I have thought the matter out for myself so as to come to a clear position as to what it all really means, and I have systematically treated *all my uterine cases during the past twenty years* in the manner here indicated, and therefore I speak of facts within my own knowledge and experience and claim a right to be heard.' The following is one of his cases – uterus retroverted, greatly enlarged; dysmenorrheoea; childlessness.

Where childlessness is the malady to be cured, the sterility being due to the womb being thick, heavy and retroverted, hysterectomy at any rate is no cure.

Surgeons are at a good deal of pains to explain to the anxious husbands that marital privileges are not barred by total hysterectomy!

The case before me now is that of a married lady, 27 years of age, two years married, and childless. I found the uterus enlarged and retroverted, which amply accounted for both dysmenorrhoea and sterility. Patient had numerous little lumps on her scalp and a lipoma on her left hip, size of an oyster; patient was also troubled with worms, was thin, and had evening flushes, and in addition to this she suffered from hay fever. Very scurfy scalp. A good deal of indigestion and moist palms. I first treated this lady's constitution for a year during which period she had *Bacillinum* (for three months), *Saw Palmetto* and *Malandrinum*, in high potencies, when she was much better in a general way but no sign of a pregnancy. I followed with *Aurum met.* in low potency which did the uterus much good; and after *Thuja* 30 and *Saw Palmetto* she fell pregnant, one year and seven months after coming to see me. A fine boy arrived in due course; and two years later a friend of hers exclaimed to me one day, 'Oh, Mrs X. has another baby!'

We shall leave the last word on this subject to the American doctor, C. M. Boger. In his little book *The Study of Materia Medica and Taking the Case* he says: 'The domain of surgery lies largely within the traumatic sphere and in the palliative, which enables the chronic patient to live, but on a lower plane. The vast majority of early operations for incipient malignancy-disease not only inflict a severe injury upon the vital force, but at least remove a suspicion only. None but the grossest materialist would do such a thing. We should use the indicated remedy from the very start, well knowing that it saves the strength of the patient and improves his chance immeasurably if an operation is finally necessary.'

CHAPTER 13

The Source of Homoeopathic Remedies

Homoeopathic remedies come from all the kingdoms – vegetable, animal and mineral. They are not purely herbal as many people believe. The following selection of names will be familiar to all; these remedies have been proved and are used regularly. I should stress that I am giving a few of the most important symptoms only under each remedy; a *materia medica* must be studied for full details.

Allium Cepa (Onion) is given to a patient with a cold displaying symptoms similar to those suffered when peeling onions! The eyes run and become red with burning and smarting; much running from the nose which is acrid, sneezing. Remember, any symptoms that the remedy can cause in a person who is well will be cured in a sick patient exhibiting similar symptoms. This is one of the remedies considered in cases of hay fever. Symptoms are all better in the open air.

Belladonna (Deadly Nightshade). The symptoms of this remedy always come on suddenly; the skin is hot and red, flushed face, glaring eyes; throbbing headache, restless sleep; throat very congested and swallowing difficult. Patient cannot bear noise, draught, touch or jar. This remedy has cured many cases of scarlet fever.

Bellis Perennis (Daisy) is the gardener's friend for it heals muscular soreness and lameness which feels as though the limb has been sprained. Joints and muscles are sore. It is excellent for complaints due to cold food and drink when the body is heated and troubles are due to cold wind.

Iris Versicolor (Blue Flag). Sick headaches are a special therapeutic field for the action of this remedy. Much burning of the throat and the whole alimentary tract. It has cured symptoms of the pancreas.

Lilium Tigrinum (Tiger Lily). This remedy has a great affinity with the pelvic organs; it has cured many cases of congestion of the uterus, prolapse and anteversion when other symptoms agree.
Ranunculus Bulbosus (Buttercup) acts on muscular tissue and skin. The walls of the chest come under its influence and it has cured intercostal rheumatism. It is one of the remedies used in the treatment of shingles.

The trees listed below are all included in our *materia medica.*
Abies Nigra (Black Spruce) has helped in dyspeptic troubles of the aged, often with constipation. Pain in the stomach always comes on after eating.
Aesculus Hippocastanum (Horse Chestnut). This is one of a group of remedies that comes to mind for cases of haemorrhoids where there is much pain and burning and the rectum feels full of small sticks.
Eucalyptus Globulus (Blue Gum Tree). This remedy is a powerful antiseptic; used in influenza and catarrh. It is indicated in relapsing fevers, acute diarrhoea and asthma when other symptoms agree.
Fraxinus Americana (White Ash) has a great affinity with the uterus and is often prescribed when the organ is enlarged; for fibrous growths, subinvolution and prolapse.
Salix Nigra (Black Willow) has a positive action on the generative organs of both sexes; symptoms are often accompanied by hysteria and nervousness.
Sambucus Nigra (Elder). The respiratory organs are often treated with this remedy. Profuse sweat accompanies many affections. Sniffles of infants and children waking up nearly suffocating also come within its sphere.

Metals play their part in healing the sick.
Argentum nitricum (Nitrate of Silver). The patient needing this remedy is fearful and nervous; impulsive, wants to do

things in a hurry; suffers from claustrophobia; has a craving for sweets. It has cleared up ulceration of the stomach.

Cuprum metallicum (Copper) has cured many cramps, especially in the calves and in the feet. It is indicated when there is spasm and constriction of the chest. When there is much nausea this remedy also comes to mind but all other symptoms must agree also.

Niccolum (Metallic Nickel). This remedy suits debilitated, nervous patients with frequent headaches (nervous, sick headaches), dyspepsia and constipation.

Plumbum Metallicum (Lead). Neuralgic pains and neuritis come within the realm of this metal, as does paralysis of single muscles. Paralysis from over-exertion of the extensor muscles in piano players. Drop-wrist.

Stannum (Tin). Its chief action is centred on the nervous system and respiratory organs; it is a very useful cough remedy when excited by laughing, singing and with copious green, sweetish expectoration.

Zincum Metallic (Zinc). When this remedy is indicated there is often trembling and twitching of various muscles and 'fidgety feet' – in continual motion.

And now we turn to minerals.

Antimonium Tartaricum (Tartrate of Antimony and Potash). Two symptoms come to mind when considering this remedy – rattling of mucus on the chest with little expectoration, and violent pains in the sacro-lumbar region – lumbago. There is much drowsiness, debility and sweat.

Borax (Borate of Sodium). There is dread of downward motion in nearly all complaints when this remedy is called for. Borax is often helpful for people who feel unwell whilst flying. Sensitivity to sudden noises is also strongly marked.

Kali Phosphoricum (Phosphate of Potassium). One of the greatest nerve remedies, especially for young people who have studied too hard. Neurasthenia, mental and physical depression are greatly helped by it. The causes of these troubles are usually excitement, overwork and worry.

Natrum Muriaticum (Chloride of Sodium – common salt). This remedy will bring comfort to many patients suffering the ill-effects of grief or fright when consolation aggravates. Tears stream down the face when coughing. If a cold begins with much sneezing this remedy will nearly always stop it developing if taken immediately.

Natrum Sulphuricum (Sulphate of Sodium – Glauber's Salt). One of the most characteristic symptoms of this remedy is 'feels every change from dry to wet weather'. Ill-effects of falls and injuries to the head followed by mental troubles.

Silicea (Silica – Pure Flint) is called for when the patient is lacking in moral or physical grit – faint-hearted, anxious. Imperfect assimilation and consequent defective nutrition. Promotes expulsion of foreign bodies from tissues.

We cannot leave out remedies from the animal kingdom.

Apis Mellifica (The Honey Bee). This remedy is often called for when oedema is present; in fact, if one thinks of the effects of the bee sting one gets a picture of some of the symptoms that *Apis* will cure – it does not matter where the swelling appears.

Cantharis (Spanish Fly) has a great effect on the urinary organs with violent paroxysms of cutting and burning in the whole renal region; painful urging to urinate. It also relieves some burns, scalds and sunburn.

Crotalus Horridus (Rattlesnake). This remedy is indicated in low septic states (think of the effects of a bite from the rattlesnake); haemorrhage, tendency to carbuncles. It has been used in the treatment of yellow fever, cholera and paralysis.

Lachesis (Surucucu Snake) is often needed in the climacteric and for patients who are very depressed and cannot bear anything tight around their throat or waist; loquacious;

jealous. It has cured many throat symptoms. The patient needing this remedy is worse after sleep.

Sepia (Inky Juice of Cuttlefish). This patient is indifferent to her family, anxious, depressed and dreads being alone. There is very often a yellow saddle across the nose. Pelvic organs are relaxed and one of the characteristic symptoms is a bearing-down sensation; wants to sit with legs crossed to support them. Limbs very restless. Sweats easily. Feels cold even in warm room.

Tarentula Cubensis (Cuban Spider). This is a remedy for septic conditions. It has helped the most severe types of inflammation where there is a purplish colour with burning and stinging pains. It soothes the patient on his death-bed, easing the last struggles.

I could fill this book with remedies but for those who are interested there are several good *materia medicas* available for further study. I have taken a handful of our remedies from the various categories of sources to illustrate their wide range, and have given only the briefest indications; in the larger and fuller *materia medicas* the symptoms of one remedy may fill as many as thirty pages.

From the foregoing you will realize that our armoury is extensive and that as long as the practitioner has the full facts, not only about the sickness but about the patient himself and how he is reacting to his symptoms, then an enormous number of cures can be accomplished.

PART TWO

Homoeopathy in Action

To demonstrate just what homoeopathy can do and the wide range of diseases that it can tackle, I am including in the next few chapters case histories taken at random from my own files, and from those of homoeopathic physicians who have done such brilliant work in the past.

It is difficult to choose from the many famous men and women who have contributed so much to this field of healing. I have decided to concentrate on British homoeopaths.

We have found that most people enjoy reading about how others have been cured and so I hope that you, too, will find the following chapters of interest.

CHAPTER 14

Cases from my own Files

A BACKWARD GIRL

Some time ago I was asked to help a backward girl of 16 years of age. She had all the appearance of being 'dull' – she came into my room, lolled in a chair, and I could get very little out of her. She did not look very clean, her hands were warm and clammy and I knew that she suffered involuntary urination at night.

I had very few symptoms and realized it was a waste of time to try and get anything more from this girl, who had come on her own. I gave her a dose of *Sulphur* 1M and asked her to come back and see me in a month's time, and I wrote to her mother to make sure that this next appointment would be kept.

When I saw her again there was quite an improvement. This time we were able to chat together and I ascertained that she got very het up anticipating events and this was one reason why she would not talk to me previously – she was in an awful panic! She also told me she felt very shy and timid, certainly a very marked symptom. I found out too that she was sensitive, moody, irritable and hated to be in a room full of people (due to her shyness, no doubt). She said she did not like anybody to fuss or console her; she often caught colds and hated cold weather, and although she was 16 years of age her menses had not yet started.

This girl needed *Lycopodium*, but as we must not prescribe it directly following *Sulphur*, I gave her an intercurrent four doses of *Tuberculinum Bov.* 200. During the following month she had a very heavy cold because of which she sneezed and blew her nose for several days; it then went down to her chest and she felt quite ill for a day or two; then she improved, and when she came to see me after four weeks she had yellow-green catarrh.

I then gave her a dose of *Lycopodium* 10M, and after two or three months she was a different person. Although she will always be rather shy and retiring she was much brighter, and her mistress at school was very pleased indeed to find that she could now study quite well, and although behind other girls for her age, she was more ready to take in what she was being taught. The incontinence at night was a very rare thing and she had no more colds. Four months after the first dose of *Lycopodium* she had another, this time in the 50M potency, and although I have not seen this girl since, I have heard from several sources that she is now quite normal; she joins in the activities of village life and has many friends. Incidentally, her menses began after the first dose of *Lycopodium*.

I doubt very much whether she would have been able to earn her own living had she not had homoeopathic treatment; she is now taking a secretarial course.

I DON'T FEEL WELL!

Mrs E., aged 44 years, came to see me complaining 'I don't feel at all well'. She told me that she had been a widow for over a year and had a great fear of cancer. An aunt had died of cancer of the rectum and a sister of cancer of the uterus; she thought her mother had died of cancer of the liver. Her mother's father had died of cancer and she thought her maternal grandmother did also. She had had a miscarriage three years previously during the third month, and had not been well since. She suffered severe aching in the right ovarian region which was worse during the first day of period (menstruation regular), and had little or no sleep because of this pain. Urination was frequent and she experienced a burning, smarting pain during and for some time after urination. She preferred cold weather. 'I'm so nervous I can hardly contain myself' was her own description, and she was constantly moving her fingers whilst talking to me. Complained that she suffered a bloated sensation in the abdomen periodically, and also some backache (sacral) and aching and soreness in the vagina.

On these symptoms I gave her a dose of *Apis* 1M.

A month later there was some improvement – much less pain in the right ovary with period. She had not been as free from it for over a year. She was given sac lac (sugar of milk given as a placebo).

A month later she complained of a dull pain low down in the vagina and weight and pressure in the stomach soon after eating; she said she had not felt so well during the past week or so.

Apis 10M was prescribed.

When I saw her four weeks later she was very much better. No pain with menses and she said, 'The last medicine helped me more than any medicines I have ever taken.' She added that she had no idea medicines could make her feel so much better.

I have had a letter since saying that she is fine.

The family history in this case was extremely serious and who can say what future trouble this medicine may prevent. *Apis* is a very deep-acting remedy which can influence the life force – I trust it will avert disease such as her relatives had suffered.

INCONTINENCE

Mrs P., aged 52, had for several years suffered from incontinence of urine for which many treatments had been tried, but still the condition persisted. She had dark hair, a sallow complexion, and was naturally morose and peevish. It appeared that the urine, which had a rather strong, pungent odour, dribbled away from the bladder almost continually each afternoon and evening, but she was quite free of this symptom during the morning. Her undergarments became saturated and she was in considerable distress.

She took *Lycopodium* 1M and was completely free of the symptom for one week, after which it began to return.

The remedy was repeated in the same potency and her symptom cleared up for three weeks, much to her delight. A further dose of *Lycopodium* 10M cleared up her trouble completely. I have seen this patient occasionally since, and now, seven years later, her incontinence has still not returned.

A CASE OF LUMBAGO

On 2 April 1961, Mrs X. came to see me as she had suffered from several bouts of 'lumbago' from time to time and her back just then was very painful. She had the first attack in 1952, the second in October 1960, and the third when she came to see me. She explained that she suffered from a sharp pain deep in the muscles of the right side of the lumbar region, with a numb feeling going down into the right nate. The pain was better on movement.

Normally one might have thought of *Rhus tox.* as 'pain better on movement', but as this was the third attack in ten years there was obviously an underlying cause and it would have been of little use to treat the superficial symptoms or the 'effect'.

A great deal of interesting information came to light upon taking the case. Mrs X. told me that she also suffered from constipation; in 1939 she had had jaundice, and measles very badly in 1942. Also, she had had pneumonia following influenza five or six years ago.

This woman had lived in the East for some time during the War, and for nearly a year in Burma she had been obliged to take Mepacrine as a prophylactic against malaria. In addition she had had six or seven smallpox vaccinations, and all the other injections one has to have when going to Eastern countries, including the one given for cholera.

I ascertained that she woke up with a metallic taste in her mouth which she said was most objectionable, and that she never felt she wanted to get up, but was all right soon after she got going. She never felt 100 per cent in the spring, and this was rather a trying time for her. She could never sit in the sun as this would make her feel sick and exhausted. She got very depressed in the damp cold, but could not stand the great heat in Burma as it was, generally, a damp heat, although she stood it better in India as this was a dry heat. She said she loved fresh air and could not sleep in a room with the windows closed. She could not endure anything tight round her neck. In the past she used to dream of falling but had not done so lately. She would weep with rage, although she would not weep easily; she disliked fuss and consolation; was anxious about things and a bit fearful – she would not like to live alone. She said she was impatient, irritable, easily offended and sensitive, particularly as to what people thought about her, as she wanted to be liked!

As Mrs X. was co-operating very well with her answers, which is not always the case, I asked her if she was jealous; she took quite a long time to answer this question and then attempted to convince me that if she was, it was not real jealousy but rather envy . . . I wrote down on my case sheet 'jealous' and underlined it! This is one of the questions that is not easily answered!

I questioned her about her food and diet – she loved salt and salty foods, bread, potatoes, sweets and cakes. I rather guessed this as she was overweight and I noticed that she had a greasy skin.

She had given me a perfect picture of *Lachesis* – worse spring; worse humid heat; worse constriction neck; jealous; anxious; angry; impatient; irritable. But the vaccinations had to be taken into consideration. In addition, you will remember that Mrs X. liked salt and salty food and had, in the past, dreamed of falling. She also told me later that she had had a collection of warts on the palm of her right hand when she was a girl. Therefore, without hesitation, I started her treatment by giving her *Thuja* – just four doses, but as she was very 'orthodox' in her outlook I knew she would not be happy with these alone and so I gave her a box of unmedicated pills to be taken twice daily.

She came to see me again on 2 May and said she felt better. Her back was improving. It ached sometimes in bed and the pain stabbed her occasionally when she was standing – but there was considerable improvement. The metallic taste in her mouth had diminished. She said she had forgotten to tell me that her nails were soft and flaking. I repeated the prescription.

On 13 June she had an excellent report to give me, saying she felt very well in herself and was enjoying walking and doing a lot of housework. Constipation still troubled her and her back still ached on turning over in bed and sometimes when sitting in a chair, but it was very greatly improved. I gave her one powder of *Lachesis* 200 and some more unmedicated pills.

About six weeks later Mrs X. wrote to say she had never felt better; there was no sign of any backache, she had plenty of energy, her constipation was much better, and she was very pleased. A friend told me some years later that she had remained well.

Although the constitutional remedy for Mrs X. was *Lachesis* I am sure the results would not have been so good had *Thuja* not been given first to clear the system of poisons left behind from the vaccinations, especially in view of the indications for *Thuja* – dreams of falling and desire for salt.

DIFFICULTY IN WALKING

On 19 November a man came to see me as he was having great difficulty in walking. He had a pain in the hip which travelled down the back of his leg to the ankle. He felt better when standing and worse when sitting, as after he had been in a chair for a little while his leg became most uncomfortable with a sensation of needles and pins. Sometimes his leg throbbed. During the War his back had become very painful; he had what the doctors called a 'slipped disc', but no treatment was given and this gradually got better. Two years before his visit to me he had had a recurrence of the same pain in his back, again travelling down his leg, and this time the doctor gave him some medicine and it cleared up, but obviously it was never cured, as some time later the pain returned. An osteopath put the back condition right but the leg-pain persisted and, naturally, the patient felt most unhappy about it. He told me that during P.T. in the War he had fallen flat on his back but otherwise he could not account for this trouble. His past history showed that he had had whooping cough as a child; he was prone to colds throughout the winter which descended to his chest, followed by yellow catarrh, which he was hardly ever without during the cold months of the year; he had had pneumonia twice. His father had suffered from pernicious anaemia and for some time a bronchial condition. One sister had polio. Patient himself detests any strong winds; loves fresh air; loathes hot, stuffy rooms as he feels overpowered in them. He takes a good deal of salt with food; is terrified of heights; very irritated by crowds of people. He has suffered with styes on his eyes during the last three years and has one wart on his hand. He used to dream of falling quite often. He worries a great deal and this makes him irritable and depressed. He would never weep normally and does not talk about his troubles; he only confides to his wife. He has a quick, bad temper. Gets very het up anticipating events. Is impatient; easily offended; very sensitive to people's feelings and rather obstinate. His troubles are left-sided. He has been vaccinated three times, the first two not taking. Had the usual inoculations during the War years. Is a very restless person and wants to be on the go all the time.

On 21 November I sent twelve powders of *Thuja* 30, one to be taken dry on the tongue at bedtime on Mondays, Wednesdays and Fridays.

On 23 December he wrote to say that he had suffered an

aggravation; for the first three or four days after starting treatment, the pain in the leg became more acute, but he slept throughout the night, which he had not done for weeks. He added that when the pain was at its height he felt as though the muscles were wound up tightly He had also had a bad head cold followed by catarrh. During the last week of treatment the pain was better, and sitting in a chair was then quite bearable.

As he was always getting colds with catarrh, and in view of the fact that he had suffered pneumonia twice and loved fresh air, I sent him, on 31 December, four doses of *Bacillinum* 200, one to be taken dry on the tongue at weekly intervals.

I heard no more until 6 February when he wrote to say he had been completely free of pain for over a month; he could sit comfortably in a chair again and felt better in every way. He said he had been working hard for long hours without distress and was sure he was cured. This has proved to be true.

CORONARY THROMBOSIS AND SMOKING

A businessman aged 46 came to see me some years ago. He had suffered from coronary thrombosis and been plagued by many boils. Of course, the heart trouble was his most serious concern, for he was happily married with two children and had a pleasant, happy disposition. He had taken the advice of his doctor and heart specialist and had been confined to bed for several weeks. The rest had allowed the damaged heart muscle to mend, but he was far from well.

On questioning him in the usual manner I discovered that he was an inveterate smoker . . . he smoked four ounces of tobacco and a large number of cigarettes each week, and inhaled all the smoke, even from the pipe. When asked how long he had done this he replied, 'All my life.' I was really horrified and knew that something drastic had to be done if he was to return to a normal life.

I had a long talk with him and in the end made him promise to give up smoking altogether and for all time, because obviously he had a tobacco heart.

I gave him *Anthracinum* 200 and *Strophanthus* 6. There was an immediate improvement – he took on a new lease of life and there has been no return of old symptoms.

HEADACHES

On 19 September, a married woman came to see me because she suffered very bad headaches. She said she knew when she was going to have a bad one as she always woke up with it, the pain being in the occiput and across her eyes. Often she vomited. On questioning, she said she hated the heat and the sun 'makes me feel ill'; wind made her very irritable. She is a chilly person – feels good in the spring; cannot bear warm stuffy rooms, and must have air; suffers from travel sickness; likes chocolate but dislikes fat, greasy food, pastries and cakes; is not thirsty; feels better at the sea; has vertigo in high places; fears crowds and cannot walk in narrow streets, feels shut in; anticipation makes her want to pass water every few minutes; had a lot of acne as a girl; cannot bear constriction round her neck; dreams constantly of trying to catch a bus or train which she just misses, and wakes up panting, with a throbbing headache. She also dreams that she is being chased; unpunctuality irritates her; she is impatient; dislikes criticism; cannot bear any noise; forgetful of names; not good at figures; bad concentration.

On 2 September she was given *Pulsatilla* 1M and sac lac.

By 16 October she felt much better, brighter and alive in the morning. Has had only one headache, on 1 October. On 7 October her right eyelid swelled up, but it went down next day. Feels much more relaxed. Her legs used to ache if she had to stand for any length of time but now she says she doesn't know she has any legs!

Gave her sac lac and asked her to report in another month.

On 22 November she wrote to say she felt very well – no headaches.

I heard about this patient through a friend several years later and she was still very well.

RHEUMATIC FEVER?

In October 1962 a friend of a patient wrote to me from southern Rhodesia saying she had no discomforts at the time of writing but frequently suffered agonizing and crippling pains in her joints. Also, 'I always cough up much mucus, generally in the mornings, and it is more marked during menses.'

Most of her troubles occurred on her left side. At the age of 11 she was suddenly struck with a burning, weakening pain in her left ankle; she had difficulty in walking home, and when the doctor came it was puffy and brick red. Subsequently she developed pains in various parts of her body and then a temperature (rheumatic fever?). Father had rheumatic fever; maternal grandmother died of T.B. of the lungs.

In 1931 patient woke one morning with severe pain in left heel. In a few days she had pains in her foot, knee, wrists and fingers, and as a result spent two months in bed – again she was said to have rheumatic fever. During both attacks she was treated with M & B and became depressed and suicidal.

Eight years ago she developed crippling pains in her right hip, but those cleared up in a comparatively short time.

In herself she is worse first thing in the morning, before breakfast. Also worse in hot summer months; she becomes enervated and often breathless. She dislikes the hot summer intensely, particularly stormy weather, but we must remember that the months before the rains in Rhodesia are called 'suicide months' as the climate is so trying. She feels full of energy in the cool weather; cannot sit in the hot sun for any length of time; feels better in fresh air; says she cannot tolerate a closed atmosphere, and if she had to sit in a warm, stuffy room she would become irritable, claustrophobic and would eventually faint. She has a great desire for sweet things (husband says she has a maniacal desire for sweets), but dislikes vinegar and cannot stand sour things; has a good appetite and usually eats biscuits between meals because she finds she gets palpitations and feels faint by the time the next meal is due if she has not had something to nibble. She is not particularly thirsty; perspires freely on exertion; loves sea air; had a few boils some years ago, also a wart and skin eruption on her back, which was quite bad for a while, during her teens; sleeps well; used to be a great worrier, but not now; is quite emotional; gets worked up when worried or anticipating events; is very sensitive.

I sent her one dose of *Sulphur* 1M to be taken dry on the tongue, and three numbered powders of sac lac to take at weekly intervals.

On 30 November she wrote and from her letter it was obvious that she was suffering from reaction as she had very loose bowel actions and an itching skin. Sent her four unmedicated powders, to be taken once weekly.

I did not hear any more until January when this patient wrote and said that nothing very much had happened, but she sent one or two more details and I dispatched *Argentum Nitricum* 30–200–IM to be taken at night, the next morning and the following night, plus three unmedicated powders.

A month later she wrote and said that she had suffered some arthritic pains and indigestion, but both had cleared up rapidly. Sent four unmedicated powders.

On 29 March she wrote saying she had had a bout of 'flu but in the last paragraph of her letter she added, 'In myself I feel cheerful – positive and more relaxed. I am sure my mind is infinitely less confused than it was and my memory much better; in fact life is good.'

Sent *Arg.nit.* 10M with three unmedicated powders to be taken at weekly intervals.

On 4 May she wrote and said she had not felt so well for a

very long time and was sure that the medicines had put an end to her aches and pains. Also the catarrh had gone. I wrote and told her to contact me should any symptoms return but I have never heard from her so conclude that she has remained well.

HOMOEOPATHY AND CHILDREN

It is always pleasing to treat a child, for we know that by taking constitutional remedies he will be strengthened and cleansed of inherited sickness, and so go forward with a clean bill of health which he will subsequently pass on to his own children.

Such a child came to me not so long ago through a friend of mine who met a very worried mother whose son was in bed with a temperature, a condition that troubled him frequently. My friend recommended homoeopathy. After an explanation the mother telephoned me for an appointment, and the following week both parents brought the boy to see me. He was a fine-looking little chap of ten, but despite this he would often be stricken, quite suddenly, with a high temperature and red throat, and would spend four or five days in bed having whatever the school doctor prescribed in the way of drugs. Gradually his symptoms would abate and he would return to his lessons, but in the course of a term he would miss quite a lot of schooling. At the age of five the boy had suffered from bronchial pneumonia and German measles, but had never contracted any other diseases.

I asked the parents about themselves. The mother was healthy and there was not much to worry about on her side of the family, but the father told me that his mother was 'chesty' and that he had been in a sanatorium for seven months with T.B. about twenty years ago. This then was the clue!

The boy himself doesn't feel too good in great heat and enjoys a cool breeze. He perspires freely on exertion; his feet sweat and the perspiration has an odour rather like rotten cheese (the boy's own description!); he has a good appetite, loves sweets and sweet things but not fat and greasy food. He is a sensitive boy and easily offended; gets worked up anticipating events and anything that he has to do in the future.

There was only one thing to do in the beginning; I gave him six doses of *Tuberculinum Bov.* 200 (three times daily for two days) plus some sac lac pills, and I asked him to come and see me again in a month's time.

I was delighted to learn that after this medicine the boy had only one slight temperature which subsided more quickly than usual, and he was not confined to bed. He had just been helping his father do some concreting which he had enjoyed, and he felt fine.

I repeated the prescription and heard no more for nearly three months, when I was told that the child was absolutely well in every way – no more temperatures, full of energy and doing well at school.

This boy had inherited a predisposition to T.B. from his father which homoeopathic *Tub.bov.* removed, changing him into a healthy, happy little person. One wonders what would have happened otherwise, but my guess is that he would have developed T.B. later on in his life just as his father had done.

CATARRH

In May a woman came to see me; she was 69 years of age and had had catarrh on and off for the past 10 years, sometimes in the form of a watery discharge, sometimes thick and yellow. At intervals she had a hard, dry cough. Her nose nearly always had a stuffed-up feeling which was worse when she sat in a draught or was ironing. When she had a cold it consistently descended to her chest. Also, she suffered slight rheumatic pains in her hands and sometimes in her toes. The left side of her neck was often a little stiff.

When I saw her she had just recovered from a second

bout of tonsillitis, but apart from this had suffered no bad illnesses – neither did she know of anything serious on either side of the family. In herself she feels limp in humid heat and her rheumatic pains are always worse in cold, damp weather, which she loathes; dry, cold weather exhilarates her; loathes warm, stuffy rooms; enjoys sitting in the sun providing she can wear dark glasses to protect her eyes from the glare; does not enjoy too much fat or too many rich foods; takes a good deal of salt; her tummy 'turns over and churns' at heights; worry and anxiety cause her to be irritable; never wants sympathy when in trouble; has a hasty temper and feels very impatient; can be irritable and very sensitive to personalities and also to music; loathes noise; does not care for anybody to see her weeping but often cries with laughter and her eyes water in strong winds; feels much better by the sea. She was vaccinated as a baby and was due to be done the next day as she was going abroad for a holiday.

First of all I gave her an antidote to the vaccination, and on 21 May she had one dose of *Natrum muriaticum* 1M and unmedicated pills to take during the month.

On 26 June she wrote to say she was feeling a little better but that she had lots of aches and pains, much more catarrh following a bad chesty cold, and now a hard cough. Sent her more unmedicated pills as she was suffering an aggravation from the *Natrum mur.*

At the end of July I heard again, and although she was much better she said she felt very tired and drained of energy. Although she could not tell me much about her family history, I felt that in view of her chesty condition following every cold (and she had many colds) her trouble would not clear up until she had some *Tuberculinum*, and I gave her four doses of the 200th potency, one to be taken once weekly at bedtime.

During the last week in August she telephoned to say she was rather alarmed – she had awakened from sleep three times during the previous ten days absolutely dripping with perspiration, and she wondered whether I could give her something to stop this. I sent her some unmedicated pills as this was a reaction from the *Tuberculinum* and I did not wish to interfere with its action.

Four weeks later she had a very different story to tell. She felt much better – the cough had cleared, the catarrh had much diminished, and she had begun to feel much more energetic; in fact, life was beginning to take on a much more rosy hue. She said that although she had had a damp eruption between her fingers several weeks ago, this had quite cleared up now. I was astonished, as this was the first I had heard about any eruption, but when questioned my patient told me that she had had outbreaks of these watery blisters between her fingers for several years and thought they were due to using detergents! As the *Natrum mur*. had caused an aggravation followed by some improvement, I decided to go back to this remedy before changing the prescription, and this time I gave her one dose of the 10M potency with unmedicated pills for a month. Once again she experienced slight aggravation, all her symptoms coming to life for a week to ten days, and then she felt a different person. She developed a good appetite, nothing seemed to worry her, she had much more energy than she had had for years.

No more medicine has been given, and although we have been through several very trying winters since, she is still feeling 'on top of the world' – messages are brought to me by her sister and various other members of her family!

DYSMENORRHOEA (PAINFUL MENSTRUATION)

A young lady from South America came to see me in April. I was told that she suffered agonies with her periods. The pains were spasmodic and much worse at the commencement, with numbness in her legs. Periods were profuse and lasted four or five days. They were clotted and sometimes dark. She suffered bad headaches during this time. She felt very het up and nervous before her period but better when the flow began. Her feet were always swollen and she had great difficulty in getting her shoes on. Her feet got very hot in bed but in winter were very cold.

Her doctor in South America told her to wind a wet towel round her abdomen to ease the pains, which it did up to a point.

I asked her about herself. She cannot sit in the sun if it is very hot; eyes water in the wind, lachrymation with laughter; likes plenty of salt; is worse for fuss and consolation; loathes fats; her bottom lip cracks; she loves the sea and says she is better when she visits the coast; she can be irritable, is easily offended, sensitive to music, and dwells on past disagreeable happenings. She had been twice vaccinated and had had one anti-diphtheria inoculation.

On 25 April I sent *Natrum mur.* 1M and unmedicated pills.

On 22 May she came to see me and said that although her last period was painful and she had fainted, she was only in bed for half a day instead of one or two days. He feet were better and not nearly so swollen. In spite of moving house and having to rush around a lot, she said she was feeling much better in herself, more energetic, and the dark rings under her eyes had gone. Gave her unmedicated pills for a month.

On 19 June she came to see me and said she was much better. She had had very little pain with her last period and the flow was not clotted as before. She told me that large red marks had appeared under the skin of her left buttock which had lasted a few days and then disappeared. Gave her more unmedicated pills for another month.

On 31 July she told me that since taking the last medicine (unmedicated pills) a circular eruption had appeared on the top of her right arm which looked like ringworm. She also had a somewhat similar eruption on her back. Her last period was not so good as it had been accompanied by quite a lot of pain. Her feet were normal and she now found her shoes too large. No headaches at all. Otherwise well. Gave her one dose *Natrum mur.* 1M and unmedicated pills for a month.

On 21 August she arrived and said that her period was much better and she had only very little pain but was now feeling lethargic and tired. The weather was very humid at the time. Gave her unmedicated pills for a month.

25 September. The girl came in looking miserable. Said she now got frightful vertigo on buses, a sensation of something in her stomach, fullness in the ears when travelling in the underground and even in a car when going uphill or down. The rash on arm and back itched just before her period. She also complained of a pain in the occiput which spread over her head to her eyes; it felt like a hammer in her head and was much worse descending in a lift. She is worse in a draught; likes plenty of clothing and bedcovers; worse wind blowing on her head; eyes still water in a wind; still worse for consolation and fuss. I gave her nine doses of *Silica* 30 – one dose three times daily for three days plus unmedicated pills for a month.

I did not hear anything more from this girl until about a year later when she brought her mother to see me. The girl apologized for not writing but said she was soon better after the last medicine and had not been conscious of her periods since; she had plenty of energy and was thoroughly enjoying life.

ASTHMA

My cousin, on returning from a business trip to Singapore, asked if I could help the chief engineer of a firm out there who was suffering from asthma. The attacks were very bad and the poor man had said, 'These will kill me in time, you know.' What a poser! Singapore is a long way away and obviously he was suffering from a very chronic condition.

However, my cousin, who is well versed in homoeopathy, brought back some interesting information about this patient.

Mr X. was 49 years of age, of a worrying temperament, a prisoner-of-war in a Japanese camp during the occupation of Malaya, where he had suffered very intensely from bad treatment and starvation. In fact the first asthma attack he had experienced was as a P.O.W. in 1943, following severe scalding of the hands. No medicine was available when this first attack came on and he suffered tightness of the chest and complete inability to expel the mucus which congested the lungs; the crisis came after 72 hours with shortness of breath and paroxysms, extreme diuresis and perspiration; any movement of the arms and legs increased symptoms. After the crisis he expectorated large lumps of what looked like cotton-wool. He recovered from this attack in 10 days and, since then, they have never been as bad because the symptoms have been controlled by drugs and he always keeps an inhaler by him. In August 1960, when this information was collected, he was nearly always breathless and would pant for breath during normal walking. Any asthma attack would usually commence in the early hours of the morning; his breathing would be noisy and his chest would feel tight and full; the inhaler would help him to expel the mucus and he would feel better by about 6 pm.

As a child, Mr X. had had double pneumonia two or three times and subsequently coughs, chest colds and occasionally bronchitis. He said he thought there was a predisposition to asthma in his medical background as his paternal grandfather had been a coalminer in Wales, and his paternal grandmother died of asthma when about 40 years of age. He was very thirsty and drank large quantities (this, of course, is not unusual in hot countries, but he consumed nine or ten cups of tea per day in addition to coffee and cold drinks). He slept heavily and got to sleep quickly providing he could breathe! He said he often dreamed that he was falling from a height off a building or tower, and added that he hated heights now, although this had not been so in the past.

In spite of the sparse information there were some clear-cut indications for *Thuja*, and so I decided it was worth while asking Mr X. some more questions. I wrote to him without delay. He replied to say that he had lived in the tropics all his working life and had lost count of the number of times he had been vaccinated against smallpox, but he added, 'It must be at least half a dozen times.' He had also had at least six inoculations against typhoid and cholera, and two or three against yellow fever. He confirmed that he got anxious and worried, often over unnecessary and trivial matters; he was very impatient, very sensitive, and because of this was easily offended – these symptoms were all strongly marked. He promised to have all his aluminium pots and pans scrapped at once and his cook-boy was told to buy some new ones of enamel or stainless steel.

On 5 December I sent him *Thuja* 30–200–1M, three powders to be taken on three consecutive nights, and some unmedicated pills for a month.

During the first week of January he wrote and enclosed a detailed report of his symptoms. His cough was about the same, his breathing better at times, but I was interested to read, 'Certainly mental and physical fatigue do not appear to be quite so apparent at the end of a working day as formerly.' It would be tedious to give a month-by-month report on this case, but suffice it to say that this patient was sent *Thuja* in ascending potencies, and at long intervals.

In February 1961 he wrote, 'I have no wheeziness in my chest; the whistles and sounds that have been with me for 18 years have ceased almost completely. My breathing is ever so much better; in fact I feel a completely new person.'

Towards the end of 1961 I heard from this patient again as he had suffered a very slight attack and his breathing was a little troublesome; as a result, I sent him *Natrum sulph.* (a complementary remedy that works well with and after

Thuja) and for three or four months I heard nothing more until a letter arrived to say he was coming to England on leave in the spring of 1963.

I saw him first on 7 May 1963 and he asked me to give him a course of treatment whilst in this country, after which he thought he could be discharged. I gave him *Lycopodium* which was indicated at the time; this caused slight aggravation – his breathing was a little difficult for a few days – but when I saw him again on 13 June he was feeling very well and enjoying his leave. He then told me he thought I ought to know that his father and grandfather had been alcoholics – he wondered whether this would have any bearing on his illness.

As one of the symptoms of asthma was 'worse at night' and in view of this last information, on 14 June I gave him a dose of *Syphilinum* 10M and hoped that this would remove any more inherited tendencies. It certainly created sharp aggravation in the form of sickness and diarrhoea almost non-stop for three days and nights, and he assured me that he could not account for this in any way; he was staying with his sister – they had eaten the same foods and she was perfectly well. After these symptoms had subsided he felt very well and his breathing was normal.

Soon after this he was obliged to have a check-up with the firm's doctor to make sure that he was fit to return to the tropics. The same doctor examined him who had seen him three years previously. On that occasion the doctor said he could not pass him as fit unless he obtained medical treatment for his chest. In July 1963 the doctor could not believe he was the same man. He measured an additional inch of chest expansion; blood pressure was normal, there were no murmurs, and generally he looked and felt very well. The doctor was told about the homoeopathic treatment and with a smile he said, 'Your homoeopath has done a very good job indeed!'

Mr X. flew back to Singapore at the beginning of August

1963 and, except for Christmas cards, I have had no more cries for help. I know he is well. My theory is that the *Syphilinum* finally purged the system of the last of its poison, and since then he has been a fit man.

APPENDIX TROUBLE?

In May 1959 a married woman aged 29 came to see me and said, 'I have a throbbing pain in the region of my appendix which is better when I am lying flat. It is not there when I get up but comes on during the day. The pain is worse when I am sitting. Food does not affect the pain but I get a lot of flatulence which I pass and bring up. I can eat anything and everything. I have had this pain for five years and I am terrified of operataions and doctors.'

I ascertained that she had suffered the usual childish complaints, but her mother told her that when very young she had had an inflamed liver. She has a sallow complexion. Otherwise she is well and has not had a cold for several years. She suffers from constipation and has no urge for stool, sometimes for two days at a time. Stools are hard and dry. She gets tired easily and her worst time is the evening when she feels very tired. She dislikes intense heat and cold and cannot sit in the sun which causes headaches and hurts her eyes. She loathes draughts and likes fresh air; hates thunderstorms and fears the dark if she is alone. She loves sweets and is very fond of salt; hates rich and greasy food and has never been able to eat breakfast, but feels very hungry around 9.30 to 10 am. She drinks seven to eight cups of tea daily. This patient fears heights and feels paralysed if forced to ascend. She is claustrophobic in a crowded room and hates crossing a busy road. She sleeps well, without dreams; is depressed when alone; bottles things up and would never in any circumstances cry in front of other people. She sometimes laughs until she cries; does not want sympathy; fears she may be taken ill. She can be impatient and indifferent to people. Comprehension is difficult.

Here I had a good many symptoms on which to prescribe, and on 9 May I gave her *Natrum muriaticum* 30, once daily for three weeks.

3 June – pain definitely better. Patient felt tired with little energy but appetite was better and there was not quite so much flatulence. Says she feels better in herself in some intangible way. Repeated the prescription.

6 July. Reported that the pain in side better. Had normal period. Has more energy and is not as constipated or depressed. No headaches. Her right foot is swollen and a red, blotchy rash appeared around her waist for two to three days. Gave her *Natrum muriaticum* 1M and placebo for a month.

21 July. Two days after last medicine had a muzzy head on and off for some days. Rash around waist reappeared on 10 July but now practically gone. Tummy uncomfortable. Has felt tired. Gave her placebo for a month.

28 August. Half-way through the month she started a cold, sneezing and watery discharge, then catarrh, yellow-green and sticky, better in the open air. Tummy better. Rash still comes and goes. Gave her *Pulsatilla* 30 night and morning for a week.

9 September. She phoned to say she felt very much better and her catarrh had cleared.

7 October. Said she had been 'up and down' so I gave her placebo for another month.

3 November. Complains of much flatulence; feels bloated. Because as a child she had inflammation of the liver, and because of many of her other symptoms, I gave her *Lycopodium* 6 three times daily for a month.

2 December. Patient said she was very much better and had more energy, did not feel so tired. From 5 November to the 23rd she had felt no pain or discomfort. Still feels nervous and slightly panicky when indoors alone but her bungalow is situated in a very lonely spot. Gave placebo for a month.

8 February. Almost cured. Only slight pain three weeks ago. No headaches. Patient is putting on weight. I gave her some *Lycopodium* 30 and told her to take it if she felt she was slipping back, but not otherwise.

27 September. Called to say that she had her old pain back again. Gave her *Lycopodium* 6 to be taken three times daily for a month.

18 November. Came in to see me saying that she felt awful, and had terrors of anticipation. Always felt hurried and must do things quickly. Fears Heights. Is worse warmth and full of fear. Without hesitation I gave her *Argentum nitricum* 200–1M–10M to be taken night, morning, night.

19 December. Better – had less pain at longer intervals and feeling better in herself. Gave her placebo.

3 February. Patient telephoned to say she was in an awful state, very nervy, and her tummy was bad again. Sent four numbered powders, the first *Argentum nitricum* 10M, the rest placebos. One powder to be taken once a week.

28 February. Wrote and said she felt very much better and able to cope. Had not felt her tummy for several days. Sent placebo.

25 March. Wrote and said she had very little pain and had passed a very good month.

In May she telephoned again and said her tummy was fine and she was feeling better in herself than she had felt for years, although she suffered a feeling of panic and palpitations in crowds, which she had on and off all her life, although for the last month it had been worse. Sent placebo for a month.

In May 1962 she called to say she was very well in every way and enjoying life to the full.

ALMOST A NERVOUS BREAKDOWN

On 10 April a young man, Mr R., aged 29, single, came to see me. He had been in the RAF, and when in Germany during the airlift had been given the very responsible job of supervising the re-fuelling of the aircraft. He would have to answer for any aircraft having to land owing to shortage of fuel. This responsibility got on his nerves to such an extent that he could not believe his own eyes, and had constantly to check and re-check what he had done. In due course he left the RAF and entered civilian life, but this state of mind got worse; for example, when driving his car he would stop every 50 yards or so to check that he had not run anybody over. He said he had a complete lack of confidence in himself.

About two months previously headaches had begun to develop which commenced with stabbing pains in his right temple; the pains would move from spot to spot in his head. Then he would suffer a pain on top of his head which grew and subsided in waves. These pains would come and go quickly.

I ascertained that he is better in the mornings, wakes easily, is more tired in the late afternoon and evening. He *hates* the cold; his hands go dead and become quite white. A room full of people makes him feel uncomfortable. He is better sitting and worse standing, the latter causing faintness. He was vaccinated once and had several inoculations in the RAF. He likes a good deal of salt, loathes rich and greasy foods and fats; gets faint missing a meal. He is fearful of heights and dislikes crowds. Had warts on his hands, some hard and some soft. Mr R. dislikes fuss, is depressed; worry and fear are always felt in his stomach, anticipation causes anxiety; he is easily offended, timid, and retiring. He likes his head well covered in bed, and dislikes a cold draught on his head. Likes to hug the fire. His skin is dry. He is tall and thin.

As the patient had a complete lack of self-confidence, was timid, retiring, worse anticipation, likes head covered in bed, worse cold draughts, easily depressed, hates the cold, hugs the fire and is worse standing, I gave him on 11 April *Silica* 1M (1 dose) and sac lac for a month.

On 8 May he came to see me; he had divided his symptoms into credits and debits. On the credit side the waves of pain in his head had gone. On 21 April he had been out in his car and had suffered no headaches. On 3 May he went for a long car journey, which in the past would have upset him, but on this occasion he suffered no headaches, he concentrated on what he was doing, and had no worries. On the debit side, for three days after taking the medicine he felt very tired, had bad headaches; then all this cleared up. He had pains in his throat, although not soreness, and he brought up much phlegm. After a few days this too cleared up. Said he was now more relaxed. Gave him sac lac for a month.

19 June. Called to see me and said his stomach was better – it does not worry him now. Did a journey of 200 miles by car and did not feel tired and had no headaches while away. When I shook hands with him on this occasion I noticed that the latter were moist and warm, and as he is tall, thin and stoop-shouldered, I asked him some further questions and ascertained this time that he is worse damp cold, standing causes weakness and he must prop himself up, must have something to eat between 10 and 11 am otherwise he feels empty; he is worse fasting, worse 11 am to 4 pm, worse draughts, suffers vertigo looking and bending down, better eating. I gave him one dose of *Sulphur* 10M and sac lac for a month.

When he came to see me again in July he said he had brought up a great deal of mucus but had been much better in himself. His odd pains had all gone. He gardened for four days and no headaches developed, and this would have been impossible before. I gave him sac lac for a month.

On 14 August he came to see me and said the last medicine (sac lac) had caused 'a snorter of a headache' for two days, after which he had felt perfectly all right. No medicine.

On 11 September he said he had had a headache yesterday and a slight one that morning which did not last. Is still bringing up quantities of mucus. He finds he gets a slight headache now when he does not get rid of any mucus. He gardens every evening which he has never done before. Gave him sac lac for a month.

16 October. Called to say he had had only one headache – still brings up much catarrh which varies, sometimes thick, sometimes watery. He now tells me that this used to burn his mouth. Generally feels very well. Gets no headaches now when driving on a long journey. Sac lac for a month.

On 6 December he called to say that headaches were a thing of the past but he still had catarrh, although not so much. Has been remarkably well and does not worry. Gave him one dose of *Sulphur* 10M (second dose) and sac lac for a month.

I heard no more of Mr R. until the following September when a relative came for treatment and told me that he remains very well indeed.

SKIN TROUBLE ON THE HANDS

In July, Mr D.W., a married man aged 45, came to see me and said he suffered from a disease which affects the palms of his hands – tiny blisters appear, they burst, and later the whole skin of each hand peels off and he has great difficulty in healing it again. The trouble started about a year ago and although it was very much better, about three weeks previously it all began again. He said he had been rather worried and had a great deal on his mind, much the same as when it had started originally. He admitted that he got very edgy at times and thought his nerves were in a bad state.

On questioning him I found that he felt better in the winter because in the summer, when he got hot, his hands would become worse. He gets irritable and restless if he sits in the sun too long. He prefers fresh air and enjoys sea air, although his hands tend to dry up and are rougher when at the coast. He is fearful of heights and of being crushed or injured in a crowd. Worry affects him, and his complaint is worse if he has any anxiety – his extremities tingle, he gets the fidgets and becomes bad-tempered. He does not like fuss or sympathy, is most impatient and always in too much of a hurry; is inclined to use wrong words when writing.

I gave him one dose of *Natrum mur.* 1M and sac lac for a month.

On 14 September I received a letter from him which said, 'From the very first week I felt very much better in myself. I had no more tense feeling, and also found I slept better and was not so irritated with the little things which used to upset me before. A friend told me that the trouble could possibly break out again and not to be worried if it did so. Just prior to my holiday my hands did start to skin again and I found that they were just a little worse whilst I was on holiday. I put this down to the fact that I had been sea-bathing and the salt water irritated them. I am pleased to say that since my return they have improved tremendously and, if they keep going as they are, I am sure they will be back to normal again. I must repeat that I feel very much better in myself and would like to thank you very much.'

Seven months later I heard that he was still very well and his hands quite normal.

BACK TROUBLE

On 2 June a young farmer, John, aged 23, came to see me and said that at the beginning of the year he had lifted a heavy weight which had put his back out. He was in hospital for three months in a plaster cast and no other treatment was given to him. When he was discharged he went to an osteopath who had given him much relief. His back gets very painful and stiff after sitting and, on rising, the first few steps give him a lot of pain and he has to grab something to prevent himself falling; after continuous movement it is better.

I did not hesitate in giving him *Rhus tox.* 30, a dose night and morning for a month.

At the end of June he wrote to say, 'I have been very

active hay-making and rock-climbing, and although I was never conscious of overdoing it, I was sometimes a bit stiff. It is better than it has ever been now. I still feel it a bit, especially after sitting for any length of time, standing still, or driving a car.' I sent him a single dose of *Rhus tox.* 1M and sac lac for a month.

On 1 July he telephoned to say there had been amazing improvement, but standing, sitting, or a day in the office causes more discomfort than an active day's farming. I sent him one dose of *Tuberculinum Bov.* 1M (as it is the chronic of *Rhus tox.*) and sac lac for a month.

In September he wrote to say his back was better but still aches sitting in the office. Sent him *Rhus tox.* 200, 1M and 10M to be taken night, morning, night, and sac lac for a month.

In October he telephoned to say that standing caused him the most discomfort, so I sent him *Sulphur* 30–200–1M to be taken night, morning, night, and sac lac for a month.

In November he came to see me with a very good report, saying he was less and less aware of his back. I gave him *Sulphur* 200, 1M, 10M to be taken night, morning and night, plus sac lac for a month.

The following February he telephoned to say that his back was almost forgotten, but he qualified this by saying he had been on holiday and not working. I sent him sac lac for a month.

In April John wrote, 'I am very pleased to say that I have almost forgotten my back. I get some soreness in my legs and back on lifting, but it goes off much quicker than it used to. In particular I can stand better and I can tackle jobs now as heavy as I've ever done in my life.' I sent *Sulphur* 50M, one dose, and sac lac for a month.

In July he reported he was quite well.

CHAPTER 15

Thomas Skinner M.D.

Thomas Skinner was one of the most brilliant British homoeopathic physicians. The story of his conversion from allopathic medicine is interesting and, in a way, unique.

Dr Clarke (*see* Chapter Sixteen) knew him well and wrote a *Biographical Sketch of Dr Skinner,* and I cannot do better than quote what he says.

It has been somewhere said that a persecuting allopath is better than an allopath who seeks to patronize homoeopathy. There are some homoeopaths who are never so happy as when an allopath bestows a patronizing smile upon them, or pats them on the back. That may do for homoeopathic individuals; but homoeopathy can no more be patronized than can the law of gravity. Both the one law and the other will work independently of any one's approval; an allopath who can look favourably on homoeopathy should not stop there; but he should become a homoeopath. There is no middle way; an honest allopath must almost of necessity be a persecutor of homoeopathy. Such was Dr Skinner until a three-years' illness had brought him to despair, and fate drove him into the arms of homoeopathy, and homoeopathy cured him. And thus it was that the honest allopath became an honest homoeopath.

Dr Skinner began his medical studies in 1849 and later became assistant to Sir James Simpson, who was most impressed by a paper written by Skinner on 'Chloroform Anaesthesia'.

Dr Clarke goes on:

Dr Skinner retained his enthusiasm for chloroform to the last; indeed, he maintained that it was as harmless as milk. And so it was in his hands. His contribution to the anaesthetic epoch was the invention of the excellent and convenient inhaler (known by his name – Skinner's Mask) and drop bottle (Skinner's Drop Bottle).

Dr Skinner went to Liverpool in 1859 and here he enjoyed a busy consulting practice for a number of years. It was during this period that he married his first wife, the daughter of a wealthy Lancashire manufacturer.

Clarke continues:

After some years, under the strain of his large practice, his health broke down and an attack of influenza which supervened left almost complete insomnia in its train. For three years he was practically *hors de combat.* At one period of the time he took a position as medical officer on board one of the transatlantic liners. After years of travel by land and sea, though his general health was greatly improved, he was in no sense cured. It was just at this time that he was incidentally 'in a very remarkable way' thrown into the arms of homoeopathy. The piquancy of the new situation will be understood when it is mentioned that hitherto Dr Skinner had been one of the most bigoted of the Liverpool allopaths and most active in passing the most delightfully thorough-paced persecuting law there is to be found in the statute book of any society. Here is Dr Skinner's own account of the state to which illness had reduced him. For three years he had been incapacitated from practice. For twenty-one months of it he had never experienced more than two hours' sleep in fourteen days, and more than once he had been as much as six weeks without knowing what it was to be one moment unconscious day or night. At the same time he was suffering from habitual constipation and terrible acidity of the stomach, for which he had taken unlimited bicarbonate of soda. His bodily and mental anguish was unutterable.

It was through correspondence about some matter apart from medicine that Dr Skinner in 1873 became acquainted with Dr Berridge; but the acquaintance led to a desire on Dr Skinner's part to know something about homoeopathy, as he had heard of some good cures when over in America. The upshot of it all was that Dr Berridge prescribed *Sulphur* for our patient in the MM potency, prepared by Boericke of Philadelphia. When Dr Skinner felt the homoeopathic remedy at work inside him it was a revelation indeed. 'I shall never forget the marvellous change which the first dose effected in a few weeks, especially the rolling away, as it were, of a dense and heavy cloud from my mind.' He was cured of the constipation, the acid dyspepsia (which he had had all his life), sleeplessness, deficient assimilation and general debility, and restored to a life of usefulness and vigour. Under the tuition of Dr Berridge he now studied homoeopathy in earnest, his textbooks being *The Organon, Materia Medica Pura, Chronic Diseases* (all by Hahnemann), and a repertory. He was advised to provide himself with two or three dozen remedies in the 30th potency, and give them whenever he felt sure he had found the similimum, but not otherwise. Thus he began to practise secretly until he had made his ground sure. He then publicly announced his changed practice and resigned his membership of the Liverpool Medical Institute to save himself from being automatically excluded by his own bylaw!

There is evidence that Dr Skinner did remarkable things with homoeopathic remedies during the succeeding years of his life. He followed the instructions of Hahnemann and the following quote from his own book is proof of how thorough he was in his learning.

'Let every man judge for himself – let him take nothing on the *ipse dixit* of any man, no, not even of Hahnemann himself, but let him examine all things well by the light that is in him, and hold fast by that which seems to him to be good and true. Let every physician and student of medicine do as I have done – carefully peruse for himself *The Organon* of Hahnemann, his *Chronic Diseases* and his *Materia Medica Pura* and I warrant him that he will rise from the perusal a wiser man. Above all, after the perusal and study thereof, let him see the practice of homoeopathy in the hands of the master in the art, and he will be forced to exclaim – have I been all this time in so great, such dense darkness, mistaking darkness for light, and light for darkness? *The Organon* of Hahnemann is the only safe and sure guide to the student of homoeopathy who desires "light, more light".'

The following are a few of his cases.

A CHRONIC CASE CURED

19 April 1880. I was called to see an elderly gentleman residing about two or three miles from my house (I then resided in Liverpool) and I had never before seen or even heard of the gentleman, and I was not at all sure whether or not I should respond to the call. It was a young servant girl who came for me in a cab, and she could not say whether her master or mistress were Homoeopathists or not. She was simply directed to bring Dr Skinner or Dr Hayward. When asked what was wrong, she said that her mistress told her to say that it was a fit of a serious kind requiring immediate assistance. Off I went in the cab, and on entering the vestibule, to my agreeable surprise, I espied a colossal bust of Samuel Hahnemann. As I knew nothing whatever of the family, it was some consolation and encouragement to think that they were admirers, and most likely believers in the Master.

When introduced to my patient, I found that he also was colossal in all his proportions; tall, very stout, bull-necked, and quite a subject for an apoplectic seizure. He lay on the floor perfectly helpless and speechless, having some control over his lower extremities and head, but none over his upper extremities, which were as completely paralysed as his tongue. His mouth was drawn to one side but I cannot say which. The hour of the attack was about 6 pm and I would be at my patient's side at about 7.30 pm. His age was about 60 years. He was neither comatose nor was his breathing stertorous, and yet there was great difficulty in getting him to understand anything – being more stupid than dazed and insensible. His pulse and heart were about normal, or if anything, hurried, and his face was flushed. I found him on a temporary bed made on the floor, and propped up somewhat with bolsters and pillows, a very wise arrangement which I did not disturb. With nothing but women in the house and only one man (myself) the bare idea of carrying 225 or 230 pounds upstairs to the bedroom, reconciled all to the existing arrangement.

Diagnosis of the remedy. This being but my second case of apoplexy with paralysis since adopting Homoeopathy, and being a total stranger to the family, I felt anything but at home, and, as the symptoms did not afford me sufficient light to enable me to decide upon the remedy, I asked a few questions of my patient's wife. I asked her if she had ever observed anything wrong with her husband's manner or state of health lately? Was he given to the inordinate use of stimulants of any kind, including much liquor? Was his temper violent, or had he given vent to a fit of rage or passion immediately before the attack, or any unusual mental or bodily excitement? Lastly, was he liable to headaches, with determination of blood to the head? To the first three questions she gave a direct negative, but to the last, she said, 'Now, doctor, you have hit it! For the last six months at least, every, or almost every, night or evening my husband has suffered a martyrdom from such headaches, and he had one of them when he dropped down paralysed and insensible.' I then asked her if she had ever noted the time when the headaches came and went? 'Yes,' she replied, 'I have invariably observed that they come at 6 pm and that my husband has generally felt better of them *before* going to bed, and that would be about 10 pm. Sometimes they have lasted an hour or more after he has been in bed.' Does his face flush when he has one, as it is now? She replied, 'Always!' Can anyone doubt the similimum in this case?

Having only a case of medicines of thirties with me, I dissolved *Lycopodium* 30 in a teacup of cold water and directed that a teaspoonful should be given every two hours until I saw him again next morning. Having some doubt as to my patient's power of deglutition, I gave the first dose myself and he swallowed it easily.

When I saw him next morning I was informed that he had passed a pleasant night, and that he had slept so naturally and so well that the attendant had only an opportunity of administering two more doses after I left. I then directed a dose to be given every four hours. After the first dose of *Lycopodium* 30 he had no more of his headaches with flushing of his face and a strong determination of blood in his head at 6 pm which he had had nightly for the last six months, and one of which he had when he was seized with his first attack of apoplexy with paralysis. Within forty-eight hours, he was able to sit up and even to converse with us, and that too at the very time when one of his evening headaches was due; and, in about six weeks, he was not only able to be up and dress himself, but the hands and arms which at the time of the attack were perfectly powerless, and all but without feeling, were so far restored that he was now able to button his shirt himself, a hitherto impossible act. With the exception of *Aesculus* 30 on one occasion, and *Pulsatilla* 30 on another, for an attack of piles, *Lycopodium* is entitled to all the credit.

CASES OF COMMON RINGWORM

At a boarding school for young ladies, in one of the healthiest neighbourhoods of Liverpool, something very like an epidemic of ringworm made its appearance, to the disquietude of the lady superintendent. The local medical man (an allopath of considerable experience) was called in, and he gave the usual full and particular directions, dietetical, cleanliness, fresh air, exercise. In spite of all his directions, dietetical, regiminal and medicinal, the mischief was not only unchecked, but it actually spread. Besides, the young ladies decidedly objected to being isolated, and, what was very natural, they began to talk to each other, and it is suspected that some of them actually wrote home to their friends.

I was totally unknown to the mistress of the school, but at the suggestion of a lady, a friend of both of us, she was induced to try what Homoeopathy could do for the malady.

The first case brought to me was Miss M., aged 16, an exceedingly fine-looking girl, of fair complexion. Her family history was strumous. She was blamed for being intellectually stupid and given to tears which are very easily excited.

On the back of her right thigh I was shown a large patch of common ringworm, *Herpes circinatus*. She told me that it itches most violently at all times, worse towards morning in bed. On being asked she informed me that she had constantly a sensation in her feet and legs as if she had on cold, damp stockings, and that she was very liable to chilblains. Menses expected every day. As soon as they are well over, she is to take a powder dry on the tongue of *Calcarea carbonica* 200 every other morning on rising.

28 October 1876, fourteen days after visit, and about one week after commencing the treatment, reports herself very much better in every respect, although the patch was still there, but paler, and itching much less. By right I should have given no more medicine, but as they resided a long way off, I repeated the *Calcarea* 200 every third morning.

17 November 1876. Steady improvement, patch all but gone; no itching; cold damp stocking sensation still present. To continue *Calcarea* 200 once a week until the appearance of the next menses, by which time the patch had entirely disappeared.

As soon as the proprietrix of the boarding school saw Miss M. improving, a batch of two or three at a time was brought to me. As it would be tedious for me and for my readers to give the details of eight or nine cases, all so much alike, I shall content myself by summarizing them.

Besides the case already given of Miss M. there were seven other cases, many of them much worse so far as the extent of the skin affection is concerned. In two of them it was on the scalp, especially bad about the edges of the hair, having all the appearance of *Porrigo scutulata,* or *Herpes* of the hairy scalp. In my views of pathology, *Herpes circinatus* and *Porrigo scutulata* are the same in cause and essence, and the one is as easy of cure as the other, without local treatment of any kind. One young lady, of exceedingly fair skin, fat and plump, and about 15 years old, had several large patches over the left breast and arm, also on the neck and thigh. I do not think that in so few patients I ever saw the disease so general over the body. With two exceptions, *Sulphur* and *Calcarea* cured every case within one month from the commencement of treatment, without isolation except that two were not allowed to occupy the same bed, whether ill or well, without change of diet, and without the simplest or the vilest local application of any kind.

It is now one year and four months since I was asked to prescribe for Miss M., and within six weeks the disease was altogether stayed and eradicated from the school. When I was consulted it was spreading.

PROLAPSUS UTERI

R. D. (coloured), who goes out to wash and iron, was sent to me by a lady friend who takes much interest in the woman. Her age is 54 and the menopause began ten years ago. She is a widow who has only had one child and three miscarriages. On 3 April 1878 she informed me that she had suffered on and off from falling down of the womb for thirty years; for the last two years she had worn a pessary, but ultimately it had to be removed on account of aggravating her misery. For the first two months it afforded relief to her symptoms. She has worn no pessary for two years.

Symptoms – she has great pain in the left iliac region and groin, worse when walking or standing, alleviated by sitting. She thinks she feels the womb return into its place when sitting. She has frequently a feeling as if she would lose the use of her left leg. She suffers from lumbar pains of a sharp shooting or cutting character, proceeding from right to left, settling down in the left groin. She has a dragging pain under the left ribs in front and to the side. The left side is her weak one, the right being altogether free. She has occasional white discharges, and she is greatly troubled with the wind. She is habitually and obstinately constipated. Hot flushes to face; subject to violent headaches of a throbbing character, and her feet are always cold and dry. Can anyone doubt the corresponding remedy?

On 3 April 1878 I gave her one dose of *Lycopodium* CM there and then, dry on her tongue, and she was to call in a week. She called when I was ill and in bed, so she called again on 15 April, complaining that ever since she saw me she had experienced aggravation of all her symptoms, especially the pain in the left groin. There was no doubt in my mind that it arose from the CM of *Lycopodium*, and be it remembered that it had lasted twelve days. I gave her one dose of the MM and on 23 April she called to say that the great bearing down and prolapse had entirely left her, but the pains in the left hypochondrium and left groin are no better. She got *Thuja* 30 night and morning until she felt better or worse.

30 April 1878 – she reported great benefit from the *Thuja*. The pain at the bottom of the left ribs is gone, the first dose affecting it, but it returned. Great pain is felt across the small of the back, and in the left groin. She got no medicine; to return in a week.

8 May 1878. The *prolapsus uteri* sensation is much less often than formerly; the bearing down is still in abeyance and the left infra mammary and inguinal pains are almost gone. No medicine.

17 July 1878. Return of the lumbar pain, the paralytic feeling in left leg, and the sensation of *prolapsus uteri*. Eructations of wind affording great relief. She got one dose of *Antimonium tart.* 1000.

24 July 1878. She reports all her symptoms are gone

again, except pain in the lumbar region, as if broken or beaten, the weak feeling in her left leg, and an occasional sense of *prolapsus*. These symptoms are worse in cold, damp weather; backache, and always wakens with her mouth parched without thirst.

She received *Nux moschata* 500, 31 July 1878. The pain in the back is greatly better, 'not nearly so racking and violent'. The weak feeling in the left leg is also much better, and is still improving. No medicine.

8 August 1878. The feeling of paralysis in the left leg is entirely gone; and the backache is much less.

17 September 1878. She feels now as if she were 'perfectly well; better than ever she felt in her life'. One month after this (17 October) she felt a return of the *prolapsus*, with an aching across the small of her back, worse in bed of a morning; she had also a red discharge with cutting pains in the hypogastrium and loins, aggravated in wet weather, and full of wind. I gave her *Carbo vegetabilis* 50M, one dose.

31 October 1878. Greatly better in all respects, and improving in health and strength.

14 November 1878. She called to return thanks and to say that she had not felt so well for years and that she is now able to do her work with comfort. I discharged her as cured, and that if ever there was a return of her symptoms she was to call or inform her friend Mrs D. As she has done neither, I feel justified in concluding that she remains well, if in the land of the living.

Comment. The only comments which I think necessary to make are: (1) This was a genuine case of *prolapsus uteri,* as I examined her and found the neck of the womb swollen and protruded fully two inches beyond the vulva. The womb was rarely more prolapsed, but she often felt as if the whole of her insides, womb and all, would come out. I did not examine her when she left me, because the bearing down was gone, which is the disease. The bearing down is the cause, the *prolapsus* the effect. Remove the cause, and the effect, the *prolapsus*, ceases. (2) I have no doubt that if I had not been in such a hurry to change the first similimum and only stuck to it throughout, I should have accomplished the cure more quickly, much more homoeopathically, and altogether much more satisfactorily so far as my own feelings are concerned. In conclusion, here is a case of *prolapsus uteri* of thirty years standing in a washerwoman cured in about seven months, without mechanical support of any kind, without local treatment, and what is most extraordinary, while she was following her laborious vocation, mostly standing. When the advocates of local treatment can show us an equal or superior success, it will be time enough for them to find fault or to ask for proof of our ability to do away entirely with local medication. No one can doubt that if this poor woman could have obtained rest and the necessities of life without standing and working for them, and having to go out in all weathers, a speedier cure might have resulted, although I think that seven months is a short time to subdue thirty years of psoric misery.

A PAIN IN THE BACK

As this case is one of the most interesting of my extraordinary cases of cure of chronic disease I give it in full.

Happening to have a colony of patients in various parts of Holland, I was invited by one of them to spend a few weeks with them, and to enjoy some splendid sport amid the wild 'long-tail' on the dunes near Haarlem. The temptation was more than I could refuse, considering that there was four square miles of the most excellent sport – say about 8000 acres.

On 28 October 1890, I took in hand the following case – Nicholas van de V., head gamekeeper to the family with whom I stayed when in Holland, aged 38, gave me the following history of his case, interpreted by one of my patients, as I scarcely know the meaning of one word of the Dutch language.

Five and a half years ago in the month of November he was watching for poachers one night in cold and wet weather. On that night he ran a great distance, and then lay down for three quarters of an hour, and when he rose, he felt a pain in his back. He went on watching and got wet through, and he got no rest until 11 am on the next day. The pain was now so bad he had to go home as soon as possible. The pain was on and off, but ultimately he was attacked by fever for which he got quinine. Since then the pain in his back has got steadily worse, relieved only by the brightness of April and May. He suffered scarcely any pain during these two months for the first two years of his illness. The locality of the pain is in the mid-lumbar region, but it gradually descended to both limbs, chiefly in the left. When bad, he feels a throbbing extending towards the navel, violent while it lasts, which is only about one minute. The blood then rushes to his head and his scalp sweats from the violence of the pain as he supposes. The general characteristic of the pain is a gnawing ache, and he says he feels as if there were a part of his spine taken out or wanting to the extent of five inches.

The time of aggravation is on awakening of a morning and at night, if awake, probably as he thinks from the warmth of the bed as the pain is somewhat relieved by getting out of bed and moving about his bedroom or sitting in a low chair with his feet as high as possible. He is in general worse if he gives way to his temper, or from a fright or other emotional causes. He is worried by trifles, which is decidedly on the increase. When sitting he experiences relief when his feet are high and close together; when standing he has relief with his fists pressing or resting on his sides, but if he leans back when standing the pain is increased; relief leaning forward.

His feet and legs up to the knees are icy cold objectively and subjectively and constantly so. After a short and quiet walk, weather permitting, they get warm, but as soon as he stops walking they return to their icy condition. In bed they are objectively warm and subjectively cold. His father died of phthisis and was subject to rheumatism for years before his death.

He has frequent faint spells without swooning, relieved by rest and slight food. As a rule he has no appetite, constant thirst with dry mouth. On awakening he has a bad taste in his mouth. He has no aversion to any particular kind of food in general – but a decided anorexia, sometimes capricious – and when he can get it he likes variety, and that not often.

His skin easily perspires – especially on the back, which is constant.

Previous to his illness he had an eruption on his hands – probably eczema or scabies – accompanied by intense itching, which was suppressed by white ointment prescribed by a physician in Haarlem, and which was made up by a chemist in said quarter which I was informed took six hours to compound.

Hebra looked upon this ointment which bears his name as a sort of 'fail me never' in the cure of eczema and which, if it did no good, it never did harm. Oh, Moses!

I know of no more powerful suppressants than the oxides and salts of lead. In this ointment we have the monoxide or litharge, or massicot, as it is called in the arts.

This ointment took a first-class Dutch 'Apotheck' six hours to compound and the sequel will give my readers the effect, Professor Hebra to the contrary notwithstanding.

The eruption had existed two months and the ointment took two months to remove the itching and the eruption. This eruption began in February 1884 and was suppressed about June of the same year, and I am informed that it was of a vesiculo-pustular and suppurative character from beginning to end – scabies?

The attack of pain from the night-watching came on in November of the same year; therefore, the burglar was shut up in the house about nine months and kept himself quiet and latent until he attempted to escape by the back door, but in doing so he threw the proper tenant on his 'beam ends'. So much for Professor Hebra and the School he so much adorns.

Treatment. I shall make short work of the treatment but I shall leave out nothing that is necessary for the enlightenment of my *confrères.*

There being no doubt in my mind that it was a case of suppressed psoric eruption, I gave my patient a single dose of *Sulphur* in high potency dissolved in a teacupful of cold water at bedtime. This was taken on 28 October 1890 and the patient was told he required no more or other medicine for a month.

23 November 1890. I was informed by letter that my patient was sleeping and eating better and on the whole was suffering less from the pain and general weakness of his back. *Sulphur* in the same high potency was repeated and sac lac was given night and morning.

13 December 1890. Complains of coldness of his legs and feet, especially in the evenings, in bed. When his feet get warm his hands get cold. Pulsations in his back. Suppressed psoric eruption after *Sulphur*. I gave him *Sepia* 50M, three doses in one day, and then sac lac night and morning.

11 January 1891. The *Sepia* removed the alternation of temperature between hands and feet and otherwise 'picked him up' greatly. He now complained of great tension and stiffness of his back, always worse in damp, cold and *foggy* weather. In order to give my readers an idea of the change for the better in my patient's health and strength since commencing treatment on 28 October 1890, I may state that in spite of the season of the year, which was always fearfully trying to him, and which generally confined him to the house, in the letter of 10 January I was informed that my patient had been out the whole day before and was not tired on returning home. He shot on that day fifty-four rabbits!

Why! two months and a half before this he was quite unable to travel beyond fifty or a hundred yards from his own lovely cottage, the property of the mistress whom he wished to serve.

The medicine now prescribed was *Baryta Carb.* 50M which afforded great relief to the tension of his back, worse in damp and foggy weather.

The *Baryta* was followed by *Calcarea* with excellent effect. *Rhus*, though strongly indicated, fell like so much water on a duck's back. During the month of October 1891, he was delighted to think he would have the pleasure of seeing me, of thanking me, and of 'walking me down'. He told his mistress, the Lady of the Manor, that 'if it had not been for your English doctor and his wee sugar pills I should have been in my grave'.

Although he is marvellously better, I do not consider him cured. I merely now report progress and I hope to be able to report still greater progress when I see him again next September or October in beloved Holland. During last October my patient accompanied a party of shooters three days a week as a *generalissimo* of the beat for pheasants, partridges, woodcock, hares and rabbits, and he seemed always the better for it, never the worse. He loves to be a hunter as much as I do. He is now upon *Silica* 1M every night and morning because the throbbing in his back and the coldness of his lower extremities, the outer sides, still continue.

THE CASE OF A DIRTY, UNMANAGEABLE BOY

As the case I am about to relate has remained well for over five years I am made to look upon it as cured.

The lad belongs to a first-class family and had the promise of a civil appointment in India, although when I was consulted he was only ten years of age. As a matter of course, unless he was cured of his dirtiness and his indifference to what others thought of him, the acceptance of the appointment was an impossibility, as his studies could not be pursued, leave alone his habits, which were intolerable in any civilized society.

A. was ten years of age when I was consulted by his parents in London on 29 December. They informed me that the master and mistress of a public boarding school had threatened to send him home, as they could not do with a boy with such filthy habits as A. The medical attendant of the school was of the opinion that medicine could be of no avail in such a case, that the boy was simply incorrigible, and deserved a good birching! The doctor at one time put it down to neglect and indifference about the motions of his bowels, and prescribed an occasional dose of 'Eno's Fruit Salts' which only made matters worse, and no more attempts at cure were made. The corporal punishment was decidedly objected to by the patient and his friends. What then was to be done? The lad must either leave the school and give up all thoughts of a lucrative appointment in India or be cured. Allopathy sung out *non possumus* – while homoeopathy held out its dove with the olive branch, and in mercy healed the youth of all his troubles, and they were many. The poor fellow was more sinned against than sinning.

On cross-examination of his mother I found that when four years old he used to pick up dung and eat it with avidity, and he was not ashamed to own up to his weakness, on the contrary, he laughed when taunted with it, so that there was no shaming him out of it. Almost his whole life he had been in the custom of constantly boring his nostrils with his fingers until they bleed. He does so still, but he used to eat what he picked from his nose. He has never been known to pass worms of any kind. He is hungry at all times, eats greedily and bolts his food; excellent digestion. He suffers from snuffles and is liable to chronic nasal catarrh every winter and spring, and he then snores loudly when asleep. All his life, or the greater part of it, he has had enlarged tonsils. The same wretched weakness showed itself in bed as well, which made the school-mistress and chamber-maids anything but friendly towards A. His schoolfellows tried to shame him by giving him all sorts of disgusting names, but his only protection was to laugh back. Hair and complexion fair, disposition fretful, easily moved to tears and decidedly mischievous. According to his mother, 'He has talent!' . . . a mother could not say less! . . . 'but is disinclined for mental work; he won't work or apply his brains in useful thought – only in mischief. He is careless and indifferent to duty and work. Good on the whole, but I never know what may happen.' The flesh struggles hard against the spirit. The mother's husband is in the church! Lastly – and this is the point on which my skill and judgment were required to be exercised – A. was continually soiling the interior of his trousers and setting up such an unconscionably unpleasant odour all round that his fellow scholars would not sit on the same form with him, nor would they even associate or play with him in the yards or on the lawn.

It was for this misfortune that the school physician prescribed 'Eno's Fruit Salts'. God forgive him! for he evidently knew not what he was doing.

29 December. I diagnosed the cause of all the boy's misfortunes, bodily, mentally and socially, to the paralysis of the sphincter ani. I do not often trouble myself about the pathology of the case; and in the present instance, although some may think that I am doing so and prescribing according to the pathology of the case, I am doing nothing of the kind. A.'s weakness or misfortune is put down as filthiness engendered or encouraged by bad habits and indifference, whereas it is due to a morbid weakness inherent in the boy's constitution. It is a disease, and not a dirty habit or vice, as ignorantly judged by his schoolmates, his masters and, shall I add, by his physician? In the first place, I have to convert the mis-named bad habit into what it really is, and the only conclusion to which I can come, is that I have a long-standing paralysis of the sphincter ani with which to deal – a

paralysis which is no part of paraplegia, nor of pyrexia, but purely idiosyncratic. Pathologists would say that it might depend upon the presence of worms, or of accumulation of faeces, or of morbid secretions, or of some morbid something irritating some portion of the mucous membrane of the ascending transverse or descending colon, or rectum, in sympathy with the sphincter ani, and thus causing it to become relaxed or contracted. So much for pathology, the only part of which worth anything is the fact that in A. the sphincter ani had long been functioning *non est*. Now for the remedy. According to my repertory, with interpolated notes, I find under paralysis of the sphincter ani *Aconite, Alcohol, Atropinum, Belladonna, Causticum, Colocynthis, Hyoscyamus, Kali Cyan, Laurocerasus, Lycopodium, Mancinella, Opium, Phosphorus, Ruta, Stramonium, Sulphur* and *Zinc.*

Sensation as if paralysed, *Coca, Sabina.*

Not feeling satisfied with any of these remedies, I had to go back to my old school experience, and in that experience, I remembered that of all the medicines having a direct control over the sphinter ani *Nux vomica* stands second to none, *Belladonna* next, and *Secale cor.* is 'not a bad third'. Of course, this is clinical observation entirely, but I never object to a well-observed clinical observation where never more than one medicine at a time is always prescribed by the observer, which was my own case as an allopath from 1854 till 1874 – twenty years. In said experience, *Nux vomica* stood at the top of the poll in paralysis of the sphincter ani; *Belladonna* in paralysis of the sphincter vesicae, especially in the incontinence of children when deeply asleep. *Nux vomica* is not in my list of remedies for paralysis of sphincter ani, but whether clinical or pathogenic, I made up my mind to commence with *Nux*, and the more so because of the determined mischievous character of A. and because he always cried like a child when asked to go to his books.

On 29 December 1881 I placed upon his tongue one dose

of *Nux Vomica* CM, and the same was to be repeated every night at bedtime until he had greater control over the sphincter ani. As my patient and his family reside more than a hundred miles from London, the greater part of my prescribing had to be accomplished by means of correspondence.

3 January 1882. His mother reports A. as much better and brighter, but the bowels are still very troublesome. Continue *Nux* another week each night at bedtime.

11 January. The bowels are decidedly less involuntary and the stools are less offensive. Stop *Nux* and let it work.

3 February. As the nasal irritation and discharge and the other symptoms of *Cina* were in the front, he received a dose of the 1M potency and the week following one dose of the 30M. The latter affected a great though temporary change for the better in his canine appetite, and the nasal discharge and irritation; so much so that the school-master and mistress were surprised at the improvement, and the doctor was chagrined when he heard of it.

27 February. As A. still had the greatest difficulty in applying his mind to his lessons and had a decided aversion to them from the impossibility of concentrating his attention to mental work, I gave him one dose of *Baryta Carb.* 50M and sac lac every alternate night.

6 April. His mother reports that he is 'a new man altogether'. 'He has complete control over his evacuations but he still cries like a child when asked to go to his lessons.' Being somewhat at a loss what to prescribe, and knowing that all the family were extremely psoric, I gave him one dose of *Sulphur* CM which was followed by an aggravation of his peevishness and sleeplessness, so I sent him *Sulphur* 2CM, one dose at bedtime. His sleep returned 'but he still weeps when asked to do anything which he does not like, especially to sit down to his lessons'. This girlish mental weakness puzzled me much and I observe in my notes of the case the following medicines which had occurred to my

mind, namely *Belladonna, Calcarea, Ignatia, Platinum, Pulsatilla, Staphisagria* and *Tarantula;* and in children *Chamomilla* and *Cina*; also from home-sickness *Phosphoric Acid.* Home-sickness was not the keynote as it was the same with A. when at home. As he now had inflammation of the gums and a bad gum-boil, and as many of his past and present symptoms were covered by *Staphisagria,* I gave him on 19 June one dose of the 20M potency to be taken at the hour of sleep. On 28 June reported very much better, and on 13 June A. 'continues quite well since last powder'.

18 August. Return of the difficulty of retaining the faeces. 'The stools pass suddenly before he is aware of it. They are green, slimy, and offensive. He snores in his sleep and suffers from nocturnal salivation.' I sent him one dose of *Nux vomica* in high potency to be taken at bedtime, and since that dose was taken 'he has not had one involuntary passage'. *N.B.* Nor has he up until now – 4 July 1887, about five years.

In conclusion I may briefly summarize the remainder of the case by stating that up until April 1886 he got an occasional dose of *Baryta carb.* 50M, the interval at first once a week, then once a fortnight, and ultimately once a month. Since 14 April 1886 he has required no medicine and has all but finished his studies at college. The tearfulness seemed to take its departure soon after the dose of *Staphisagria.*

On looking through my notes I failed to have recorded a very curious incident in the case of this rather remarkable youth, A. He was a great coward, and like most cowards, he was fond of striking those younger than himself, and even dumb animals. A. took a fiendish dislike to a noble and quiet, inoffensive dog, the property of the school-master, and he was more than once found in the back yard beating and kicking this poor animal. When asked the reason why, he could give no reason for the action. As A. was in consequence threatened with expulsion from the school, his mother appealed to me, and not in vain. I sent *Belladonna*

20M, one dose at bedtime, dry on the tongue. A. has never since 'assaulted others' younger than himself, and the dog and he became excellent friends.

THE BORDERLAND OF INSANITY

In November 1886 I was consulted by a gushing young Irishman of a thoroughly go-ahead disposition, barring a decided tendency to very severe headaches and nervousness. He has had them on and off for as long as his mother can remember, and his age is fifteen. During the last four years they have become worse, and somewhat changed in character. They are now *worse on waking*, increasing as the day advances; he becomes sick and retches until he goes to sleep. The retching is aggravated by the least movement and it is accompanied by a deadly nausea and giddiness. He also at times suffers from a dull, stupid, drowsy headache. All the head symptoms are relieved by sleep which is not readily get-at-able. The location is both sides of the head and vertex, and of a shooting character from side to side.

I learned from his mother that he had been under the care of a well-known physician who 'practises homoeopathically' in the West of England. His prescription is a remarkably good example of homoeopathics. His diagnosis was: 'My good lady, your son's headaches are arising from a peculiar state of his stomach and blood, bringing about a condition of general anaemia. His assimilation is also all wrong and I think it is traceable to *a want of salt in his system*. Encourage him to take *plenty of salt* with his meals.'

The boy was fond of salt and took more than enough already in his meals, but having received the sanction of a physician he went in for it until he actually craved salt, and when his mother consulted me, she and the lad stated that he partook of it freely whenever he could get the chance.

The boy was directed to drop the salt altogether, and I placed upon his tongue *Natrum muriaticum* CM. In the course of about a month he was free of headaches and constipation. Some will say that the cure affected by the CM potency was much more likely due to the removal of the cause, the abuse of common salt, ordered by the doctor. It must not be forgotten that the headaches and constipation existed almost all his life, that is before the doctor's prescription, and they were only made worse by it. One thing is certain, *the aggravation in the morning on awakening* was a feature unknown to the patient before the doctor's isopathic prescription, and it was the first symptom or condition of the headaches which disappeared, clearly pointing to the CM as the factor. In fact, after that one dose he never had another headache *on awaking*. Headache on awaking is all but characteristic of *Natrum muriaticum*.

I was now introduced to a new phase of my patient's medical eccentricities, and the wonder to me was that I was not informed at first of what now follows.

28 April 1887. Ever since the sudden death of his father some five or six years ago, he had been subject to *great nervousness when out walking alone*. The young man is fearless on horseback or when driving, and he prefers a restive and lively to a quiet animal – yet, for all that, very frequently when out taking a constitutional by himself, more especially on a quiet country road, he will be seized suddenly with horror, an awful dread or fear comes over him. He literally is compelled to stand still, as he cannot move a limb – and if he can move, he is compelled to race home as fast as his limbs will carry him, as he feels that he is being pursued by some horrid thing and he dare not turn round to look. This occurs in open day.

If headaches and constipation were more than a match for the West of England homoeopathic physician, this nervousness fairly made him cave in. By way of consolation to the widow, she was informed that they would gradually disappear as he grew older. In other words, he would grow out of them. The spirited young fellow informed me that so great was the fear and feeling that he was actually pursued by some fiend, 'he would knock any man down who tried to stop him'.

When I come across a proving by Hahnemann, whether found or 'not found' by the learned Dr Richard Hughes, what a confidence it inspires me with. In the *Chronic Diseases*, I read recently under the moral symptoms of *Anacardium Orientale, 'When walking, he felt anxious as if someone were pursuing him. He suspected everything around him.'* Having no higher attenuation than the 1M I gave him seven powders. One to be taken at bedtime and one with or after every nervous attack.

30 June 1887. Greatly better in every respect, has only required to take three of the seven powders of *Anacardium*. He has never again required to 'run home because of being pursued by an imaginary foe'.

10 April 1888. I was consulted again because of extreme nervousness *when about to undergo a journey by rail*. He is then seized by a severe *tremor of the hands and a cold clammy sweat breaks out all over him*. He feels himself to be hopeless, unmanned. The strangest and perhaps the most inexplicable part of his nervousness is the fact that he becomes *all right as soon as he is in the train*. He is similarly unmanned when almost anything is expected of him. I gave him about twenty doses of *Arsenicum album* 1M, one to be taken at night at bedtime and no more unless the feeling returned, when he was to take a dose with every return.

7 March 1889. He had had no return.

A CASE OF CONSTIPATION

By the recommendation of Dr A. Spiers Alexander of Plymouth, Devonshire, I was consulted with regard to a case of constipation of the most confirmed character, extending over the lifetime of a young lady of twenty years of age.

I give Dr Alexander's history of the case:

First seen on 14 November 1890.

1. Five years ago had an attack of perityphlitis.

2. Ever since then she has suffered from constant pain in right iliac fossa, radiating upward and across abdomen. She also frequently gets more severe and spasmodic attacks of pain in the same region coming and going suddenly and lasting for half an hour. These pains leave her intensely prostrate for days.

3. Since the perityphlitis she has been obstinately constipated – more so than ever before – the bowels being perfectly torpid and no action or inclination for stool without aperients and enemata.

4. Constant nausea and often bilious.

When the young lady came under my care, the following was the photo which I took of her case – the gist of it:

Appetite indifferent, thirst capricious, prefers very cold water or else very hot – so hot, she says, she likes to drink it boiling out of the kettle in a tumbler (these are her own words, oft repeated); taste slimy before breakfast now and again, and breakfast is her best meal; sinking, empty, exhausted feeling at the epigastrium daily at 10 am, 3 pm, 6 pm and 7 pm, relief at 8 pm; right ovarian pain, a full heavy ache shooting from right to left, worse ascending, rising from lying or sitting, carriage exercise on rough roads or anything that shakes her; always aggravated on the first day of her menses; the duration of this pain has lasted upward of three years, and it followed an attack of peritonitis in 1888.

Her chief complaint is habitual constipation, but since 1888 there has been no inclination for stool; the bowels and rectum seem perfectly torpid or paralysed. The stools are hard, large, dry like rubble and occasionally in round balls, passed with the greatest difficulty, and only with the aid of aperients and enemata. There has been marked recession of the stool since January 1888.

The medicines more particularly indicated in this case are plainly *Silica, Sulphur, Lycopodium, Opium, Plumbagum,*

Nux, Bryonia, Sepia, Magnesia mur., and *Pulsatilla.* I give them in the order of their homoeopathicity in my mind.

1 April 1891. I prescribed *Silica* CM dry on the tongue, and another dose at bedtime on the same day followed by the usual placebo.

6 April 1891. No change, repeat *Silica* CM, a dose every night at bedtime until the bowels respond naturally.

13 April 1891. No change one way or the other. *Bryonia* CM, a dose at bedtime every night and morning if constipated.

8 May 1891. *Bryonia* did neither good nor harm. Prescribed *Lycopodium* 10M every night and morning, and at 3 pm unless better or worse as regards the constipation.

15 May 1891. *Lycopodium*, like *Bryonia,* did neither good nor harm. As all those carefully selected remedies had failed, I gave my patient an intercurrent dose of *Sulphur* 10M. This was followed by no improvement, although it may have paved the way for something better. The medicines now running through my mind were *Sanicula, Calcarea, Natrum mur., Aqua marina* and *Opium.* As the young lady resided in the neighbourhood of the sea I next prescribed, on 27 May, *Aqua marina* 20M, a remedy which has cured dozens of cases of seaside constipation in a single dose. She was directed to take a dose every night, or night and morning if constipated.

4 July. *Aqua marina* affected the constipation the same as so much water on a duck's back. I now prescribed *Opium* 50M followed by *Opium* CM, both in single and repeated doses, but without the slightest effect.

I was now but at my wits' end, and my patient and her mother and friend's patience and faith were well nigh exhausted, when a happy thought struck me. I remembered a case which I saw with my revered friend, the late distinguished Hahnemannian, Professor H. N. Guernsey, when I had the honour of visiting him in Philadelphia in 1876. The case looked very much like *Magnesia mur.*, but *Mag.*

mur. failed *in toto. Alumen* 45M cured the constipation and all else. The *Alumen* was prescribed by Professor Guernsey alone, after I left Philadelphia.

On 1 August of this year I prescribed *Alumen* 1M to my patient to be taken in one dose every night at bedtime, or night and morning if constipation was unaffected by the nightly dose.

23 August 1891. I received the following letter, the patient residing over 200 miles from me:

'Dear Dr Skinner. A great improvement has taken place in my daughter's condition. The bowels have lost their torpor, and now with a little injection of tepid water she is able to feel a natural relief. The pain in the side is much better. The medicine has suited her well.'

29 August 1891. I gave her sac lac until our next meeting which occurred about a fortnight later. Mother and daughter called at my rooms in London and the expression on their countenances at once told me that all was more than well. They overwhelmed me with thanks because, as they said, *all* A.'s symptoms had disappeared as if by magic.

I gave a few globules of *Alumen* 1M, but on no account was a single dose to be taken unless the constipation returned.

Remarks. 30 September 1891. My patient remains perfectly well in every respect. What cured the patient? Was it the *Silica* or any of the previous carefully and judiciously selected remedies, coming into action? So far as my own judgment is concerned, I would as soon believe that the moon was made of cream cheese as to believe in any such absurdity. The *Alumen* acted at once and has continued to act without a single repetition since 23 August 1891.

In conclusion I have much pleasure in quoting Dr H. N. Guernsey's work, edited by his son Dr Joseph Guernsey, of Philadelphia, and before doing so, I beg leave to honour the illustrious dead in stating that since the days of Hahnemann and Bonninghausen there has been no greater Hahnemannian than the late Dr H. N. Guernsey. He writes:

'I have been led to the use of *Alumen* (Common Alum) quite extensively in a variety of ailments characterized by *a most obstinate constipation which has been existing for a long time.* Some years ago a lady came to me suffering from very violent attacks of gastralgia, attended with nausea, vomiting, retching, etc., and unable to bear the least nourishment for ten days together. She also had most obstinate constipation; the bowels moved once in ten days; faeces dry, hard, black, sometimes large, sometimes like sheep dung, and voided with the greatest difficulty. *Alumen* 45M in a few days made her bowels regular and natural, and for several years she had no return of her gastralgia. She still keeps *Alumen* by her and at the first sign of the constipation she takes a few pellets, one dose, and it is all-sufficient. From a thin, spare, weakly woman, she has become plump and hearty.'

CHAPTER 16

Dr John Henry Clarke

Another interesting homoeopathic physician is John Henry Clarke, who died in the 1930s. He wrote a number of books, but his monumental work is the *Dictionary of Practical Maria Medica* in three volumes which is widely used today.

Dr Robert Cooper, another homoeopath, organized a dining club in which he, Dr Compton Burnett (*see* next chapter), Dr Skinner and Dr Clarke would dine together regularly and discuss their cases. Dr Clarke filled over 100 notebooks taking down all the interesting facts about remedies and case histories. Much of this information is included in his Dictionary, which took him over fourteen years to complete.

For many years Dr Clarke visited his patients in a horse-drawn carriage. I am told that this was rather like an office inside, as the good doctor never lost an opportunity of working on his books. My late partner, Noel Puddephatt, knew Dr Clarke well, and used to tell how his bulldog sat in his consulting-room, quietly watching what was going on!

It is interesting to note that while Dr Skinner always used high potencies, most of Dr Clarke's patients were given low ones.

NASAL POLYPUS

A year or two ago I was consulted by letter on behalf of a young lady, aged 20, in the country, who had been troubled for three or four years with an excessive discharge from the nose and dropping of discharge from the back of the nose down the throat. The least cold air aggravated the complaint and, conversely, it was better in a warm room. She suffered, in addition, from cold, damp feet; faint feelings, and bilious sick headaches.

She received *Calcarea* in very high potencies at rare intervals. From the first the symptoms began to improve. Later on, *Thuja* was given and afterwards *Dulcamara, Silica* and *Stannum*, her health and the local symptoms steadily improving all the time. About eighteen months from the commencement of the course she passed from her nose a polypus an inch and a half in length. The passing was preceded and followed by sharp bleeding. There has been no recurrence since.

It may be objected that the treatment occupied a long time, whereas an operation could have relieved the patient in a few minutes. This is true so far as the removal of the polypus is concerned, but the effect of the medicinal treatment was to bring about a complete constitutional change in the patient, and to work a constitutional cure. Polypi have an awkward habit of recurring after removal by operation; but when a cure is wrought by medicine the tendency to recur is removed. Moreover, operative removal of a polypus does not cure the original irritation which gave rise to the formation as constitutional treatment does.

FISTULA

Mrs M. R., aged 38, had consulted me occasionally for several years on account of constipation (for which she had previously taken Liquorice powder twice a week), piles and other troubles, which had been entirely relieved by *Sepia* and other medicines. I had not seen her for four months when she came to me on 22 October 1892. Ten days before she had had a swelling on the right side of the anus, with very great pain at times, of a pricking, shooting character, and bleeding. The lump had gone on to the formation of an abscess and had discharged, and the discharge still continued. If the discharge ceased for a time, the patient felt ill and low-spirited. There was a pile on the right side, and on the same side a hard nodule, in the centre of which was the opening of a fistula.

She had *Silica* 3 four times daily.

14 November. Has been much better. She had a new swelling on the other side but was better after it. This appeared on 8 November and disappeared entirely without discharging. Has had a good deal of discharge at times from the opening – sometimes mattery, sometimes blood. Has a sensation as if something were lodged in the bowel.

I gave her one dose of *Sepia* 30. This kept her right till the following March.

11 March 1893. Mrs M. R. has had influenza and bronchitis and the cough had caused the fistula to open up again. She was suffering from a scaly eruption on the face, acidity, indigestion and pain about the abdomen from left to right after eating, and constipation.

She had *Sarsaparilla* in a high potency.

25 March. This patient called to see me and told me her bowels were acting better; the fistula was much better but the rash on her face was not so well; she had pains in the hypogastrium and under the left shoulder-blade.

She now received a course of medicines, *Alumen* 30, *Sulphur* 30, and *Psorinum* 30, given in succession in that order with very great relief, in which the first-named medicine seemed to have the principal share.

In June there was some return, and the same course proved effective.

On 12 October Mrs M.R. again had some difficulty in passing a motion, with bleeding, and a sensation that the passage was closing up. A local practitioner had strongly urged her to have an operation.

I gave her *Sepia* 30 and *Natrum mur.* 30 on alternate weeks.

There has been no return of the old trouble, as I have ascertained from the patient, who called upon me years afterwards about something else.

With regard to the rash on her face, I may mention that Mrs M. R. discovered she always had it after drinking Indian tea. China tea did not produce the same effect.

INFLAMED GLANDS IN BOTH AXILLAE

Miss T., aged 22, consulted me on 24 October 1892. She had been away in Scotland, which was her home, and had returned on 1 September. She then had a swelling under the left arm. This was lanced by a medical man about the end of the month and discharged a good deal. Now the lump had returned and was painful and tender. She felt tired; had a sinking feeling from 10 to 11 am; suffered from constipation with haemorrhage at times; had cold feet, inclined to be damp; was drowsy and heavy in the day-time. She was worse in damp weather and better in cold, frosty weather.

She received *Hepar* 6 four times a day and the abscess soon opened spontaneously and rapidly healed. Afterwards, boils appeared on the left arm.

She had *Sulphur* 30 and afterwards *Nitric acid* 30 and got quite well, and I did not see her again until the following February.

On 3 February she told me she had a cold for a week with influenza pains about her. During the same time she suffered from pains under her right arm where I found two abscesses – one the size of a bean, the other no larger than a pea. She had taken *Sulphur* on her own account. I now gave her *Hepar* 6.

22 March. Miss T. said her right arm got quite well, but five days ago a little pimple developed in her left armpit which broke. There is now a swollen gland but the pain is not in the gland – it is in the site of the little pimple. There is not much itching in connection with this; there was when the left axillary glands were inflamed before.

I gave her *Rhus tox.* 30 and she has had no more trouble with her arm since.

TEA DYSPEPSIA

Emma E., aged 39, a dressmaker, consulted me at the London Homoeopathic Hospital on 21 June 1883, complaining of the following symptoms – great nervousness; pain in the left side when she ate; sensation as if there was a weight on her shoulders and back, especially when tired; aching in the nape of the neck all day; her breath was offensive, her gums used to bleed and she had a bad taste in her mouth with white tongue; her sleep was restless. The bowels were regular and appetite good. She took her meals at regular intervals and drank nine cups of tea during the day.

I told her she must give up her tea and gave her *Merc. sol.* 6 in drop doses four times daily.

She returned in a fortnight and reported that she had reduced her allowance to six cups of tea daily.

The sharp pains she complained of were better than they had been for years, and she slept better; the breath was still offensive. I repeated the same medicine.

She was not able to attend for a few weeks and having been out of medicine was not so well. She was so very nervous. By this time she had got down to four cups of tea each day. I again repeated the medicine.

On 11 August she received *Act. rac.* for headache and did not return until 6 October when she reported that the medicine had done her head good, but now she had soreness of the chest and much flatulence. I gave her *Carbo veg.* 6, one drop four times a day.

On 3 November Emma said she had kept well till today. Now has palpitation; headache at the back of the head, sore feeling within the head; giddiness and flatulence. I gave her *Gelsemium*, one drop to be taken four times daily.

On 17 November, a fortnight later, she reported that she had not been so well for years. Her head was very much better and she had hardly any palpitation. She had now brought herself to two cups of tea daily. She received more of the medicine and soon after ceased to attend.

In each instance the medicine given responded admirably to its indications, but I question if she would have received much benefit if she had not, besides, cut down her allowance of tea. It is possible to antidote a poison when the poison is being taken but it is easier to antidote its effect when it is no longer present. Sometimes the effects of a poison, if not antidoted, will last for years after the last dose has been taken.

DYSPEPSIA RESULTING FROM NERVOUS DEBILITY

A youth called John with the above history consulted me a year or so ago for his indigestion. He had great flatulence, which he was continually belching, acidity, heartburn, great sleepiness (which was a serious trouble to him, as he was working for an examination). He had queer feelings in his head, and had attacks of nausea, but did not vomit. His bowels were constipated. He came from a dyspeptic family, and he had been allowed to eat indigestible things when a child, but that was not the cause of his present attack, though both circumstances helped to make it the difficult case it was to treat.

There were certain things that made his symptoms worse. The eructations were worse after eating water-melon or rice pudding, and much worse after blanc-mange and custard.

He had a voracious appetite.

I put him on a very strict regimen which he faithfully followed. He had been in the habit of dining in the middle of the day and taking tea in the afternoon about four hours after dinner, and a supper late. I told him to take only three meals a day, at 8.30, 1 o'clock and 6.30. He was never to eat as much as he could; he was to take no tea or stimulants of any kind, but to drink, for breakfast, milk with boiling water, take only a very light meal in the middle of the day of beef or mutton with vegetables (excluding potatoes) and some milk pudding; a similar meal was to be taken at 6.30

and nothing after or between. For breakfast I allowed him bacon with stale bread, toast or biscuit. After the last meal he was not to study but to read light things and take a two-mile walk before going to bed.

Then I cut down his sleeping hours. He had been sleeping too much, from about 10.30 to 7.30. I ordered him to be in bed at 10.45 and to rise at 6.45, take a cold sponge-bath and work before breakfast.

Under this regimen he made considerable improvement, but the chief features of his indigestion remained unchanged.

Nux vom. gave him a great deal of help and *Nux moschata* did something towards relieving the drowsiness. *Acid phos.* lx, five drops in water for a beverage to be drunk at lunch and dinner, also proved helpful. *Calc. carb.* and *Pulsatilla* relieved the acidity and finally *Natrum mur.* completed the cure, relieving constipation as well as the other remaining symptoms of indigestion.

He was altogether under treatment about ten months. At the end of this time he was able to work many hours a day without feeling any drowsiness, and he won a scholarship.

CHAPTER 17

Dr James Compton Burnett

Dr Burnett is remembered as one of the great homoeopaths. He was related to the writer Ivy Compton Burnett and was an uncle of Dr Margery Blackie (physician to the Queen), although he died before she was born. He was another allopath who eventually became dissatisfied with allopathic medicine.

Dr Burnett is reputed to have rediscovered the stinging nettle – *Urtica urens* – the use of which in gravel and urinary affections goes back a long way. Burnett used it a great deal in diseases of the spleen (he wrote a book on this subject) and found that patients to whom he gave it often passed quantities of gravel. But he learned of another application for *Urtica urens* in a somewhat surprising way. One of his patients sent for him while suffering from malaria. He prescribed several medicines for her and heard no more for several weeks, when she visited him in his consulting-rooms. 'How are you, Mrs X.?' he asked. 'I am glad the medicines cleared up your fever.' 'It was nothing to do with your medicines,' replied Mrs X. 'I made no headway at all, and when my charwoman came in to clean for me and saw how ill I was she recommended that I drink stinging-nettle tea, and that put me right.' This led Burnett to experiment, and subsequently *Urtica urens* became his favoured prescription in cases of fevers of the East.

Willingness to pursue treatment recommended by a charwoman shows the greatness of this man's character.

SEVERE INTERCOSTAL NEURALGIA OF SEVEN YEARS' DURATION

Mrs C. J., 62 years of age, came under my observation

on 26 November 1890 for a terrible neuralgia of the left side of the trunk, just behind the spleen and the base of the left lung. The pain was most severe and described as of a screwing character. During the past seven years the patient had been going from one doctor to another, and finally on this day came to me most unwillingly and in sheer despair, driven hither by a severe attack then on. These attacks were not well defined as to time, but they were distinctly intermittent, and started as a small pain, going on *crescendo* and eventually passing off *decrescendo*. Mrs C. J. had been vaccinated three times; and moreover she tells me she once had true cow-pox, caught from a cow. She has travelled a great deal around the world, and though very strong she has had a great many diseases which included measles, whooping cough, chicken-pox, scarlet fever, South American fever (ague cured by Quinine), yellow fever, jaundice and rheumatic fever. All things considered I was of the opinion that it was a malarial splenalgia, and so prescribed *Urtica urens* (mother tincture), 10 drops in water three times daily.

16 December. My patient told me she had one attack of pain; appetite much better. 'The medicine roused me and made me tremble.' She looks quite a different woman.

16 January 1891. Mrs C. J. has had no attack and considers herself quite cured. 'I am also not so cold and do not feel the cold so much as I did.'

There was no further attack of neuralgia until the month of November 1891. This was, however, not very severe, and the same remedy in half the dose was quickly efficacious. Then in July 1892 there was a threatening again but it came to nothing, and there has been no further return of the neuralgia whatsoever.

I name this in the headline Intercostal Neuralgia because that was what her numerous other physicians had treated her for. My own conception of the nature of the case is expressed in the name Malarial Splenalgia.

MISSHAPEN HEAD: ADULT MENTAL INFANCY OF A MAN TWENTY-SEVEN YEARS OF AGE

Mr J. B., big in stature, aged 27, was put under my treatment in May 1889 by his relatives on the strength of my opinion that he might be rendered more or less normal by medicinal treatment, notwithstanding the fact that he was 27 years of age and still mentally infantile. Looking at him full in the face one noticed his forehead was very bulging; no eyelashes; a dull expression; general head-form abnormal. The history is that of 'water in the head as a child' and that he has never been 'like others'; his sisters say 'he is soft' and call him 'daft'. Being unable to do any head-work he has had none to do but has remained mentally fallow, and hence, though the son of gentlefolk, is quite illiterate. The skin of his head seems to him to be very 'tight' (most probably a physical fact primarily due to the watery state of the encephalon), whereof he complains a good deal; also of pain both in his forehead and at the back; his skin is very dusky; a number of his symptoms are aggravated at night.

I examined him closely and roused his interest in his own case. He was in no sense insane, but clearly had plenty of mind; but it was hidden behind a cloud. He would seize his scalp in his hands and tell me impressively that it was too tight, and he complained of being such a heavy sleeper, and of not being able to do anything at figures or any head-work.

I call very special attention to this case because it fully illustrates my contention that lying mentally fallow is not the proper treatment for juvenile cephalic invalids. This young man, being the son of gentlefolks of means, position and intelligence, was allowed to lie mentally fallow all his life on medical advice and he certainly grew up all right except for his dunderheadedness. Not only so, but he had an outdoor life, and when a full-grown man he was, on advice, sent to a colony with a very bracing, invigorating climate to rough it, and he carried out the things so completely that he worked for long hours at heavy, rough outdoor work, quite getting his own living at felling timber and heavy farm-work; it considerably strengthened his body, but he, at the time of which I am writing, had just returned from his long absence 'roughing it' as dunderheaded as he ever was. Now note the effect of treatment.

The first remedy that I gave him was *Lueticum* in very high potency which was followed by an 'irritation of hands and face that keeps him awake by night; it burns; does not trouble him by day'. His head is better.

Thuja 30 followed and seemed to try him a good deal. He had been vaccinated twice.

He then had *Nux vomica* and after that *Bacillinum*, and here he began to learn arithmetic, his head being so much better; and in September the first prescription was repeated.

23 October. Getting quite strong; pigeon-breastedness much less pronounced. He is getting on well with his learning the 'three R's'.

Gave him *Morbillinum* 30.

27 November. He is now enjoying his learning, principally writing and arithmetic.

Bacillinum, Zincum acet., Thuja and *Calc. phos.* carried us on to the year 1891, when my patient had so far progressed in his learning that he obtained a berth in a city financier's office where he still continues earning his living at head-work entirely.

The foregoing case very aptly illustrates the thesis which I am here trying to maintain, viz. that it does not suffice to leave the delicate and backward in a fallow condition trusting to their 'growing out' of their maladive conditions, for they are nearly as likely to grow into them as to grow out of them. This young man remained mentally fallow as far as learning was concerned and he made no mental progress. His muscles were used for these were well exercised; his brain did not improve, for it lay fallow. It was allowed to lie fallow because it was unfit for work, and no doubt it was wise not to work it in its unfit state; but that did not suffice.

You cannot grow a good biceps by carrying your arm in a sling, neither can you cultivate brain-power by leaving the brain idle. Muscle power is gained by muscular exercise; brain power is gained by brain exercise. And if the brain is in a morbid state, the malady from which it is suffering must be cured, whereafter the brain may be safely exercised and thereby strengthened. Muscle exercise does not directly strengthen the brain, neither does brain exercise strengthen the muscles; due exercise of each duly develops each; over-exercise of either is at the cost of the other. A given organism can produce only so much and no more. Great brain-workers are not muscular; great muscle-workers are not at the same time capable of great brain-work; it is impossible, all cackle to the contrary notwithstanding.

RHEUMATIC ENDOCARDITIS IN THE COURSE OF RHEUMATIC FEVER

I was fetched one day in February (17th) 1879 by a gentleman in the City to see his wife, a lady of about 55 to 60 who was lying dangerously ill at the end of the third week of rheumatic fever. This gentleman, who is an old homoeopath of thirty years' standing, and whose knowledge of remedies and disease is really remarkable for a layman, had treated the patient himself, and with no inconsiderable success considering the severity of the case, but suddenly his wife's condition became very alarming on account of the rheumatism having apparently seized the heart. I found this condition: patient was propped up in bed and breathing very rapidly; the lips bluish; tongue dry and coated; anxious expression of face; puffy under the eyes; moist rales all over chest; no appetite at all, could just suck a grape or sip tea; profuse perspiration; limbs swelled and painful, the joints almost as firmly locked as if anchylosed, cannot move hand or foot for pain and from this swelled, inflamed state of the joints; flesh of hands puffy; bones of hands swelled, almost immovable and tender.

I ordered *Aurum foliatum*, second trituration, very frequently. This was to be given along with no auxiliaries.

Why did I order *Aurum*? Because it affects the heart and respiration very much like they were affected in this patient and because it moreover produces profuse perspiration, profound weakness, anorexia and great anxiety. Then the bones were greatly affected.

18 February. A little easier. Repeat medicine.

19 February. Better in all respects. Repeat medicine.

20 February. Considerable improvement in the action of the heart; breathing comfortable; so out of danger. Repeat medicine.

22 February. Continued improvement. Repeat medicine.

24 February. Quite comfortable. Continue the *Aurum* and to have *Nat. sulph.* 6 in alternation with it. My reason for alternating was that I thought it imprudent to leave off the Gold and yet *Nat. sulph.* was now indicated.

2 March. My patient is sitting by the fire. Appetite good.

6 March. Heart, joints, bones and hands free from rheumatism; is sitting by the fire quite comfortably; appetite good; tongue moist but slightly furred; feet swell a little towards evening.

This is going to press and hence I cannot give the sequel (delay at the printer's enables me to say that patient's recovery is complete; she is now quite well) but this case so well illustrates the action of Gold on the organic tissue of the heart that I here insert it.

When I saw the patient first I gave a bad prognosis, and had it not been for Gold I fear it would have been realized. Auxiliaries did not do it, for I used none; faith in the doctor did not cure her for the patient had never seen me before.

POSTSCRIPT

Homoeopathy and the Royal Family

This is being written during the celebrations of the Silver Jubilee of Queen Elizabeth II. In September 1952, a few months after her accession, Her Majesty bestowed her patronage on The Royal London Homoeopathic Hospital. But we must delve a little into recent history, for members of the Royal Family have been treated homoeopathically for many years. Some say Queen Victoria was the first 'royal' to be interested in homoeopathy, but we know that King George VI (father of our present Queen) was converted as a young man. He was a sailor-prince and had suffered badly from sea-sickness since childhood. No doctor could find a cure until somebody suggested that homoeopathy might hold the answer. Dr John Weir prescribed the most similar homoeopathic remedy and it worked! Dr Weir was associated with the Royal Family from 1923 when he became physician to the Duke of Windsor (then Prince of Wales). From 1928 until 1953 he was physician to King George VI and Queen Mary, his mother.

Having been cured of sea-sickness the late King, then Duke of York, began to take a great interest in homoeopathy and to make a study of it. He prescribed many remedies for himself and his family when they suffered minor ailments. It was only natural that his wife, Queen Elizabeth (the Queen Mother), should share his interest and that their two daughters, Princess Elizabeth and Princess Margaret, should have homoeopathic treatment when they were ill. He introduced homoeopathy to his mother, Queen Mary, and to his brother, the Duke of Gloucester, who became Patron of the Homoeopathic Research and Educational Trust.

King George VI was Patron of The Royal London Homoeopathic Hospital from 1920 (when he was Duke of York) until he died. On the occasion of the centenary of the hospital he sent a letter to the chairman in which he said:

I have now been personally associated with The Royal London Homoeopathic Hospital for a quarter of a century and am therefore especially glad to join in the celebrations of the hospital's centenary.

To all connected with it I send my sincere congratulations, with the earnest hope that it may long maintain its record of achievement.

The Queen has continued her father's interest in homoeopathy and paid her first visit to the Hospital in 1955, an occasion to honour the 200th anniversary of Samuel Hahnemann. She was given a unique bouquet comprising 42 flowers used in the preparation of homoeopathic medicines. The first thing the Queen did was to visit Sir John Weir who was in bed in a private room recovering from a fall. The Queen asked him how he was progressing and added with a smile, 'You are in very good hands, sir.'

In April 1960 a dinner was held at the Savoy Hotel in London, an occasion to mark Sir John's 50 years as a homoeopathic physician. Telegrams were received from the Queen and also the Queen Mother, who said, 'His skill and kindness to so many will never be forgotten.' (After the King's death Sir John became physician to the Queen Mother.) This function was attended by the Duke and Duchess of Gloucester – their interest in homoeopathy never waned, and they generously attended many homoeopathic functions. Sir John Weir was renowned for his fund of anecdotes, and when making his after-dinner speech he mentioned that on one occasion Queen Mary had visited the hospital and left some flowers with him. Later he took them up to the children's ward and asked a small cockney boy if he knew who had sent them. He didn't know, and when Sir John told him it was Queen Mary the boy replied, 'Blimey, how did she know I was here?'

When the Queen and the Queen Mother travel abroad they have a box of first-aid remedies with them and these, we know, are frequently used. Princess Margaret and the Prince of Wales also have their first-aid kits and use *Arnica* whenever necessary. Homoeopathic remedies are supplied to the Royal family by A. Nelson & Co. Ltd, homoeopathic chemists in London who hold the Royal Appointment to the Queen and to the Queen Mother.

When Sir John Weir retired the Queen appointed Dr Margery Blackie in his place. This made history as she was the first woman to be in the Royal team of doctors. The present Duke of Gloucester has taken over his late father's position as Patron of the Homoeopathic and Educational Trust because he too has proved for himself that homoeopathy works.

The Queen in her Jubilee year is having little rest or relaxation. She has agreed to all the exacting schedules and in some has even added extra commitments. Those around her say she knows exactly how much she can do, which to an onlooker is a good deal more than most, and I feel sure that homoeopathy contributes in great measure to her good health and stamina.

Glossary of Medical Terms

Acrid	Pungent; irritating
Alimentary canal	The tube through which food passes from mouth to anus
Anchylosis	The growing together of two bones
Articular	Relating to the joints; articulation of the skeleton is the way in which bones are joined together
Callosities	Circumscribed areas of thickened skin due to friction or pressure
Callous	New bone formed when a fractured bone unites
Chancre	Syphilitic ulcer
Climacteric	Change of life
Coccyx	The last bone of the vertebral column
Congenital	Existing at birth
Constitutional	Relating to the total individuality of the patient
Contused	Bruised; an injury when the skin is not broken
Coryza	Inflammation of mucous membranes of the nose usually marked by sneezing
Costive	Constipated
Diuresis	Excessive excretion of urine
Dysmenorrhoea	Difficult and painful menses
Epigastrium	The region in front of the stomach
Eructations	Belching
Erythema	Red patches on the skin
Euthanasia	A painless or calm death
Excoriation	Abrasion of the skin
Expectoration	Ejection of mucus from the mouth

Extensor	A muscle which extends or stretches a limb
Faeces	The refuse material expelled from the bowels through the anus
Fauces	The short passage between the back of the mouth and the pharynx
Fibroids	Matter composed of fibrous tissue
Fibrous	Containing fibres
Fistula	A long, narrow suppurating canal
Gagging	Retching
Herpetiformis	Resembling herpes
Hysterectomy	Excision of the uterus
Incipient	Beginning, initial
Incubus	A person or thing that oppresses like a nightmare
Inspiration	The drawing in of breath
Intercostal	Between the ribs
Laceration	A tear
Lachrymation	Excess of tears
Lesion	An alteration, structural or functional, due to injury
Leucorrhoea	Discharge between monthly periods
Lipoma	A fatty tumour
Lumbar	Pertaining to the region of the loins
Lupus vulgaris	A tuberculous disease of the skin
Malignant	Virulent, threatening life
Mammary	Pertaining to the female breast
Menses	Monthly periods
Miasm	Hahnemann's word for the basis of all disease
Morbid	Pertaining to disease or diseased products
Nape	Back of neck
Nosode	A remedy made from disease products
Occipital	Pertaining to the back of the head
Oedema	Dropsical swelling

Pancreas	A long, flat gland behind the stomach
Parotid	Situated near the ear; e.g. the parotid gland
Paroxysm	A spasm; a sudden increase in intensity of existing symptoms
Pathological	Dealing with the nature of disease
Pedunculated	On a little stalk
Pelvis	The bony basin composed of the hips, and the lower bones of the spine, and holding the bowels, bladder and organs of generation
Pemphigus	Crops of pustules
Periosteum	Membrane covering bone
Placebo	Unmedicated substance prescribed to keep patient happy when no medicine is required
Plethoric	Fullness of blood
Polypus	Tumour arising from a mucous surface
Potency	Strength
Primal	First in order of time
Prolapse	The falling or sinking down of the part
Psora	The original constitutional defect
Puberty	The period when reproduction first becomes possible
Renal	An index of symptoms
Repertory	Pertaining to the kidneys
Retention	Retaining or holding back, e.g. the holding of urine in the bladder
Retroversion	Tilted or turned backward, as in retroverted uterus
Rigor	Stiffening or rigidity of muscle
Roseola	A rosy-coloured eruption
Scabies	A contagious skin disease
Sentient	Capable of feeling
Similimum	The most similar remedy
Sinus	A hollow cavity

Splenalgia	A pain in the spleen
Strumous	Affected with scrofulous tumour
Subinvolution	Imperfect involution of the uterus after delivery
Sycosis	The miasm based on the venereal disease gonorrhoea
Tendon	A band of dense, fibrous tissue forming the termination of a muscle and attaching it to the bone
Traumatic	Pertaining to or caused by an injury
Vertex	Top of head
Vitiating	Spoiling; lessening the efficiency

APPENDIX A

Homoeopathic Hospitals in the National Health Scheme

THE ROYAL LONDON HOMOEOPATHIC HOSPITAL
Great Ormond Street, London WC1N 3HR.
Tel. 01-837 3091

GLASGOW HOMOEOPATHIC HOSPITAL
1000 Great Western Road, Glasgow G12. Tel. 332 0382

GLASGOW HOMOEOPATHIC HOSPITAL FOR CHILDREN
221 Hamilton Road, Glasgow G32. Tel. 778 1185

GLASGOW HOMOEOPATHIC OUT-PATIENT DEPARTMENT
5 Lynedoch Crescent, Glasgow 3. Tel. Douglas 4490

THE MOSSLEY HILL HOSPITAL – In-patients
Park Avenue, Mossley Hill, Liverpool. Tel. 051-724 2335

THE LIVERPOOL CLINIC
The Department of Homoeopathic Medicine
1 Myrtle Street, Liverpool L7 7DE (Out-patients)
Tel. 051-709 5475

BRISTOL HOMOEOPATHIC HOSPITAL
Cotham, Bristol 6. Tel. Bristol 33068-9

TUNBRIDGE WELLS HOMOEOPATHIC HOSPITAL
Church Road, Tunbridge Wells, Kent. Tel. 0892 26111

APPENDIX B

Homoeopathic Chemists

AINSWORTHS HOMOEOPATHIC PHARMACY
38 New Cavendish Street, London W1M 7LH.
Tel. 01 935 5330, or, 01 486 0459.

FREEMAN'S PHARMACEUTICAL & HOMOEOPATHIC CHEMISTS
7 Eaglesham Road, Clarkston, Glasgow. Tel. 041-644 1165.

THE GALEN PHARMACY (J. A. EILES, MPS), HOMOEOPATHIC & DISPENSING CHEMISTS
1 South Terrace, South Street, Dorchester, Dorset.
Tel. Dorchester 3996.

E. GOULD & SON LTD, HOMOEOPATHIC CHEMISTS
67 Moorgate, London EC2. Tel. 01-606 5359.

KILBURN CHEMISTS LTD, HOMOEOPATHIC AND DISPENSING CHEMISTS
216 Belsize Road, London NW6. Tel. 01-328 1030.

NELSON'S
73 Duke Street, Grosvenor Square, London W1M 6BY.
Tel. 01-629 3118.

All these pharmacies will send by post.

APPENDIX C

One Hundred Remedies with their Common Names

Aconitum napellus	Aconite
Actea Racemosa	Black Snake-root
Aesculus hippocastanum	Horse chestnut
Agaracus muscarius	Toadstool
Allium cepa	Red onion
Aloe	Aloes
Alumen	Common potash alum
Alumina	Oxide of Aluminium
Ammonium muriaticum	Sal ammoniac
Anacardium	Marking nut
Anthracinum	Anthrax poison
Antimonium tartaricum	Tartrate of Antimony and Potash
Apis mellifica	Honey bee
Arnica montana	Leopard's bane
Arsenicum album	Arsenic trioxide
Baptisia	Wild indigo
Baryta carbonica	Carbonate of baryta
Belladonna	Deadly nightshade
Bellis Perennis	Daisy
Borax	Borate of sodium
Bryonia	Wild hops
Calcarea carbonica	Carbonate of lime
Calcarea phosphorica	Phosphate of lime
Calendula officinalis	Marigold
Camphor	Camphor
Cantharis	Spanish fly
Capsicum	Cayenne pepper
Carbo vegetabilis	Vegetable charcoal
Caulophyllum	Blue cohosh

Causticum	Hahnemann's *Tinctura acris sine Kali*
Chamomilla	German chamomile
China	*Cinchona officinalis* – Peruvian bark
Chromium kali sulphuratum	Chrome alum
Cocculus	Indian cockle
Coffea	Coffee – unroasted
Colchicum	Meadow saffron
Colocynth	Bitter cucumber
Conium	Poison hemlock
Cuprum metallicum	Copper
Dioscorea villosa	Wild yam
Drosera	Sundew
Dulcamara	Bitter-sweet
Eupatorium perfoliatum	Thoroughwort
Euphrasia	Eyebright
Ferrum phosphoricum	Phosphate of iron
Fluoricum acidum	Hydrofluoric acid
Gelsemium	Yellow jasmine
Glonoine	Nitro-glycerine
Gnaphalium	Old Balsam
Graphites	Plumbago
Gunpowder	Gunpowder
Hamamelis Virginica	Witch hazel
Hepar sulphuric calcareum	Hahnemann's Calcium sulphide
Hydrastic	Golden sea
Hypericum	St John's wort
Ignatia	St Ignatius bean
Ipecacuanha	Ipecac – root
Iris versicolor	Blue flag
Jaborandi	*Pilocarpus pinnatifolius*
Kali bichromicum	Bichromate of potash
Kali carbonicum	Carbonate of potassium
Kali phosphoricum	Phosphate of potassium
Ledum	Marsh tea

Lycopodium	Club moss
Magnesia carbonica	Carbonate of magnesia
Magnesia muriatica	Muriate of magnesia
Magnesia phosphorica	Phosphate of magnesia
Mercurius corrosivus	Corrosive sublimate
Mercurius hydrargyrum	Quicksilver
Millefolium	Yarrow
Natrum carbonicum	Carbonate of sodium
Natrum muriaticum	Chloride of sodium (salt)
Natrum sulphuricum	Glauber's salt
Nitricum acidum	Nitric acid
Nux vomica	Poison nut
Onosmodium	False Gromwell
Petroleum	Crude rock oil
Phosphoricum acidum	Phosphoric acid
Podophyllum	May apple
Psorinum	Scabies vesicle
Pulsatilla	Wind Flower
Rhododendron	Snow rose
Rhus toxicodendron	Poison ivy
Rumex crispis	Yellow dock
Ruta graveolens	Rue-bitterwort
Sabadilla	Cevadilla seed
Sabina	Savine
Sanguinaria	Blood root
Sepia	Inky juice of cuttlefish
Silica	Pure flint
Spongia tosta	Roasted sponge
Staphysagria	Stavesacre
Sulphur	Sublimated sulphur
Symphytum	Comfrey – knitbone
Tabacum	Tobacco
Tamus	Black Bryony
Tarantula cubensis	Cuban spider
Thuja occidentalis	*Arbor vitae*
Urtinca urens	Stinging nettle
Verbascum	Mullein

Bibliography

ARNICA, THE WONDER HERB, Phyllis Speight, Health Science Press.

BEFORE CALLING THE DOCTOR, Phyllis Speight, Health Science Press.

CHILDREN'S TYPES, Dr D. Borland, British Homoeopathic Association.

CHRONIC DISEASES, Dr S. Hahnemann, Boericke & Tafel Inc.

CHRONIC MIASMS, Dr J. H. Allen, Boericke & Tafel Inc.

CLINICAL REPERTORY, Dr J. H. Clarke, Health Science Press.

COMPARISON OF THE CHRONIC MIASMS, Phyllis Speight, Health Science Press.

CONDENSED MATERIA MEDICA, Dr C. Hering, Boericke & Tafel Inc.

DICTIONARY OF PRACTICAL MATERIA MEDICA (three vols), Dr J. H. Clarke, Health Science Press.

DOMESTIC PHYSICIAN, Dr C. Hering, Boericke & Tafel Inc.

DRAINAGE IN HOMOEOPATHY, Dr E. A. Maury, Health Science Press.

ENCYCLOPAEDIA OF PURE MATERIA MEDICA (ten vols), Dr T. F. Allen, Boericke & Tafel Inc.

ESSENTIALS OF HOMOEOPATHIC PRESCRIBING, Dr H. Fergie Woods, Health Science Press.

GUIDING SYMPTOMS (ten vols), Dr C. Hering, Boericke & Tafel Inc.

HOMOEOPATHIC DRUG PICTURES, Dr M. L. Tyler, Health Science Press.

HOMOEOPATHY FOR THE FIRST-AIDER, Dr D. Shepherd, Health Science Press.

HOMOEOPATHY IN EPIDEMIC DISEASES, Dr D. Shepherd, Health Science Press.

HOMOEOPATHIC MATERIA MEDICA WITH REPERTORY, Dr W. Boericke, Boericke & Runyon Inc.

HOW TO TAKE THE CASE, Dr E. B. Nash, Boericke & Tafel Inc.

HOW TO USE THE REPERTORY, Dr G. I. Bidwell, Health Science Press.

INTRODUCTION TO THE PRINCIPLES AND PRACTICE OF HOMOEOPATHY, Drs Wheeler & Kenyon, Health Science Press.

KEYNOTES AND CHARACTERISTICS OF THE LEADING REMEDIES, Dr H. C. Allen, Boericke & Tafel Inc.

LEADERS IN HOMOEOPATHIC THERAPEUTICS, Dr E. B. Nash, Boericke & Tafel Inc.

LECTURES ON HOMOEOPATHIC MATERIA MEDICA, Dr J. T. Kent, Boericke & Tafel Inc.

LECTURES ON HOMOEOPATHIC PHILOSOPHY, Dr J. T. Kent, Ehrhart & Karl Inc.

THE MAGIC OF THE MINIMUM DOSE, Dr D. Shepherd, Health Science Press.

MANUAL OF PHARMACODYNAMICS, Dr R. Hughes, Leath & Ross.

MATERIA MEDICA PURA, Dr S. Hahnemann, Homoeopathic Publishing Co. Ltd.

MORE MAGIC OF THE MINIMUM DOSE, Dr D. Shepherd, Health Science Press.

NEW REMEDIES, Dr J. T. Kent, Ehrhart & Karl Inc.

THE ORGANON, Dr S. Hahnemann, Boericke & Tafel Inc.

OVERCOMING RHEUMATISM AND ARTHRITIS, Phyllis Speight, Health Science Press.

THE PATIENT, NOT THE CURE, Dr M. Blackie, Macdonald & Jane's.

PHYSICIAN'S POSY, Dr D. Shepherd, Health Science Press.

POINTERS TO COMMON REMEDIES 1 to 9, Dr M. L. Tyler, British Homoeopathic Association.

PRESCRIBER, Dr J. H. Clarke, Health Science Press.

PRINCIPLES AND ART OF CURE BY HOMOEOPATHY, Dr H. A. Roberts, Health Science Press.

PUDDEPHATT'S PRIMERS, N. Puddephatt, Health Science Press.

REPERTORY TO HOMOEOPATHIC MATERIA MEDICA, Dr J. T. Kent, Ehrhart & Karl Inc.

SENSATIONS AS IF, Dr H. A. Roberts, Boericke & Tafel Inc.

SIGNPOSTS TO HOMOEOPATHIC REMEDIES, N. Puddephatt & M. Kincaid Smith, Health Science Press.

TESTIMONY OF THE CLINIC, Dr E. B. Nash, Boericke & Tafel Inc.

THE TREATMENT OF CATS BY HOMOEOPATHY, K. Sheppard, Health Science Press.

THE TREATMENT OF DOGS BY HOMOEOPATHY, K. Sheppard, Health Science Press.

THE TREATMENT OF HORSES BY HOMOEOPATHY, G. Macleod, Health Science Press.

VACCINOSIS, Dr J. C. Burnett, Health Science Press.

Index

W H BATES, M.D.

BETTER EYESIGHT WITHOUT GLASSES

THE CLASSIC METHOD OF RETRAINING THE EYES.

Most people who wear glasses needn't. The simple, regular exercises of the Bates Method retrain eyes that have come to rely on glasses – that have become 'lazy'. The Bates Method is a series of exercises that first relax the eye muscles and then retrain them to focus efficiently and without strain. The explanations are simple and the Method easy to follow.

Its most famous exponent was the author Aldous Huxley who could barely see even to read the book: 'Within a couple of months I was reading without spectacles and, what was better still, without strain and fatigue.'

This is a revised edition of a book that first appeared in 1919: the Bates Method has been proved a success over and over again ever since. No-one with eye-trouble can afford to ignore it.

'Better Eyesight Without Glasses could be the most helpful reprint of the year'
Bookseller

£1.95

YOGA AND YOUR HEALTH
SONYA RICHMOND

Yoga and Your Health deals with the Yoga of the physical body – Hatha Yoga – and shows how its practice can give successful protection against the stresses of modern life. Hatha Yoga works on the simple principle that, in order to function on a higher level, the first step must always be to rid the body of the impurities that cause illness and impede spiritual development.

Illustrated

95p

YOGA MADE EASY
DESMOND DUNNE

Desmond Dunne is the Principal of the Insight School of Yoga. He has adapted the ancient Asian discipline of Yoga to the twentieth century Western way of living, and includes chapters on:

- The Yoga way to banish nervous tension
- Health-giving postures and rhythms
- The Yoga way to strengthen internal organs
- How to improve your sleep
- The Yoga way to enjoy good digestion

Illustrated

£1.50